OPTICAL COHERENCE TOMOGRAPHY

Edited by **Masanori Kawasaki**

Optical Coherence Tomography
http://dx.doi.org/10.5772/56293
Edited by Masanori Kawasaki

Contributors
Martine Mauget-Faÿsse, Benjamin Wolff, Alexandre Matet, Vivien Vasseur, José-Alain Sahel, Hironori Kitabata, Takashi Akasaka, Michael Leitner, Alexandra Nemeth, Elisabeth Leiss-Holzinger, Karin Wiesauer, Günther Hannesschläger, Robert James Lowe, Ronald Concetto Gentile, Nadiya Al Kharousi, Bettina Heise, Stefan E. Schausberger, David Stifter, Carl Arndt, Shinichi Yoshimura, Masanori Kawasaki

Published by InTech
Janeza Trdine 9, 51000 Rijeka, Croatia

Publishing Process Manager Iva Simcic
Technical Editor InTech DTP team
Cover InTech Design team

Additional hard copies can be obtained from orders@intechopen.com

Optical Coherence Tomography, Edited by Masanori Kawasaki
p. cm.
ISBN 978-953-51-1032-3

For EU product safety concerns:
IN TECH d.o.o., Prolaz Marije Krucifikse Kozulić 3, 51000 Rijeka, Croatia, info@intechopen.com or visit our website at intechopen.com.

Meet the editor

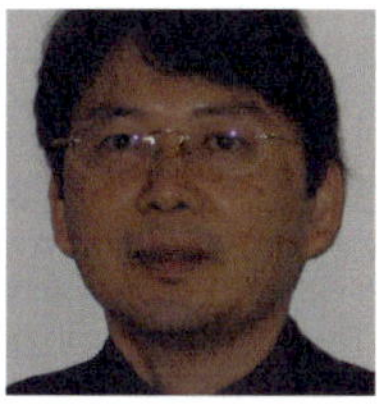

Dr. Masanori Kawasaki is a Senior Lecturer of Department of Cardiology, Gifu University Graduate School of Medicine. He received his MD and PhD from Gifu University Graduate School of Medicine. He developed a unique technique for tissue characterization of coronary plaques as an integrated backscatter intravascular ultrasound (IB-IVUS). After completing clinical training in cardiology in Japan, he conducted research on optical coherence tomography in Wellman Laboratory of Photomedicine, Harvard Medical School as a Research Fellow. After coming back to Japan, he has conducted many researches on cardiovascular imaging.

Contents

Preface IX

Section 1 Ophthalmology 1

Chapter 1 **Current Applications of Optical Coherence Tomography in Ophthalmology 3**
Nadia Al Kharousi, Upender K. Wali and Sitara Azeem

Chapter 2 **B-Scan and 'En-Face'Spectral-Domain Optical Coherence Tomography Imaging for the Diagnosis and Follow-Up of White Dot Syndromes 33**
Benjamin Wolff, Alexandre Matet, Vivien Vasseur, José-Alain Sahel and Martine Mauget-Faÿsse

Chapter 3 **Application of Optical Coherence Tomography and Macular Holes in Ophthalmology 49**
Robert J. Lowe and Ronald C. Gentile

Chapter 4 **Optical Coherence Tomography in Neuro-Ophthalmology 77**
Tony Garcia, Ghislain Bonnay, Ayman Tourbah and Carl Arndt

Section 2 Atherosclerosis 101

Chapter 5 **Visualization of Plaque Neovascularization by OCT 103**
Hironori Kitabata and Takashi Akasaka

Chapter 6 **Optical Coherence Tomography (OCT): A New Imaging Tool During Carotid Artery Stenting 117**
Shinichi Yoshimura, Masanori Kawasaki, Kiyofumi Yamada, Arihiro Hattori, Kazuhiko Nishigaki, Shinya Minatoguchi and Toru Iwama

Chapter 7 **Optical Coherence Tomography for Coronary Artery Plaques – A Comparison with Intravascular Ultrasound 127**
Kawasaki Masanori

Section 3 Engineering 137

Chapter 8 **Full Field Optical Coherence Microscopy: Imaging and Image Processing for Micro-Material Research Applications 139**
Bettina Heise, Stefan Schausberger and David Stifter

Chapter 9 **Optical Coherence Tomography – Applications in Non-Destructive Testing and Evaluation 163**
Alexandra Nemeth, Günther Hannesschläger, Elisabeth Leiss-Holzinger, Karin Wiesauer and Michael Leitner

Preface

In 1991, optical coherence tomography (OCT) was initially introduced to image the transparent tissue of eyes at a level of resolution significantly greater than conventional ultrasound technique. OCT uses infrared light to produce images on a micrometer scale. The intensity of the reflected light is displayed as a false color or grey scale image. OCT imaging is analogous to ultrasound B mode imaging, except that it performs imaging by measuring the intensity of reflected or back scattered light rather than acoustic waves. An optical beam is scanned across the tissue and material, and the reflected light is measured as a function of depth and transverse position.

Preliminary clinical studies in ophthalmology have demonstrated that OCT can non-invasively image the retina with high resolution and should be a powerful diagnostic tool for a range of macular diseases. Then, OCT was applied to many fields of medicine and engineering such as oncology and cardiology. This book is intended to serve as up-to-date knowledge of this technique, not only for medical doctors and students but also for researchers and engineers. Contents of this book were divided four sections: ophthalmology, oncology, atherosclerosis and engineering. It is our hope that this book will provide readers with comprehensive information of OCT.

Finally, I wish to give special thanks to all the contributing authors and the extraordinary staff of the open access publisher InTech, in particular Ms. Iva Simcic and Ms. Ivona Lovric, for their tireless supports.

Masanori Kawasaki, MD, PhD, FACC, FJCC
Senior Lecturer of Department of Cardiology
Gifu University Graduate School of Medicine
Japan

Section 1

Ophthalmology

Chapter 1

Current Applications of Optical Coherence Tomography in Ophthalmology

Nadia Al Kharousi, Upender K. Wali and
Sitara Azeem

Additional information is available at the end of the chapter

http://dx.doi.org/10.5772/53961

1. Introduction

Optical coherence tomography (OCT) was first reported in 1991 as a non-invasive, cross-sectional ocular imaging technology (Huang et al., 1991) and today is the most promising non-contact, high resolution tomographic and biomicroscopic imaging device in ophthalmology. It is a computerized instrument structured on the principle of low-coherence interferometry (Huang et al., 1991; Hrynchak & Simpson., 2007) generating a pseudo-color representation of the tissue structures, based on the intensity of light returning from the scanned tissue. This noninvasive, noncontact and quick imaging technique has revolutionized modern ophthalmology practice. The current applications of OCT have been improvised and expanded dramatically in precision and specificity in clinical medicine and industrial applications. In medicine, the technique has been compared to an in-vivo optical biopsy. As the resolution of OCT has been improving with time, the localization and quantification of the tissues has accordingly, become more refined, faster and predictable (Ryan SJ, 2006). What was initially and mainly a posterior segment procedure, OCT has now wider applications in anterior segment of the eye as well. The first anterior segment OCT (AS-OCT) was available in 1994. Its current use in cornea and refractive surgery including phakic intraocular lens implantation, laser-assisted in situ keratomileusis (LASIK) enhancement, lamellar keratoplasty and intraoperative OCT has opened promising therapeutic and diagnostic options in both research and clinical applications in ophthalmology. With an improved scan speed and resolution, the new models of spectral-domain (SD)-OCT allow measurements with an even lower variability (Leung et al., 2009). Due to reduced measurement errors, e.g. due to motion artifacts, the precision to track and interpret tissues has increased sharply (Leung et al., 2011). OCT is intended for use as a diagnostic device to aid in the detection and management of ocular diseases, however, it is not intended to be used as the sole aid for the diagnosis. Ultra-high resolution (UHR) OCT is a new imaging system that is being used in several clinical and research purposes. It is an objective technique and has been used for evaluation of tear fluid dynamics, contact lens fitting, imaging of corneal structures, and to describe the characteristics of epithelium, stroma and Descemet's membrane in corneal dystrophies and degenerations (Wang et al., 2010; Shen et al., 2010; Shousha et al., 2010]

2. The machine

There are different models of OCT machine available in the market. This chapter is based on observations made with Cirrus-high definition (HD) spectral domain (SD) OCT (Carl Zeiss Meditech Inc., Dublin, CA; software version 4.0). The light source of OCT is a broadband superluminescent diode laser with a central wavelength of 840 nm. This light generates back-reflections from different intraretinal depths represented by different wavelengths. The acquisition rate of Cirrus-HD-OCT is 27 000 A-scans /second. The axial and transverse resolutions are 15 and 5 μm, respectively. The vast increase in scan speed makes it possible to acquire three-dimensional data sets. Current OCT models are mainly designed for analysis of optic nerve head (optic disc cube), macula and anterior segment of the eye. The tomograms are stored on the computer and/or archive medium, and can be quantitatively analyzed. A CCD video monitors the external eye and assists with scan alignment, while a line scanning ophthalmoscope provides a clear image of the tissue addressed by the scan.

The main hardware components of the OCT include the scan acquisition optics, the interferometer, the spectrometer, the system computer and video monitor. Before scanning the patient looks into the imaging aperture and sees a green star-shaped target against a black background (Figure 1). When scanning stars, the background changes to a bright flickering red, and the patient may see thin bright lines of light, which is the scan beam moving across the field of view. Normally, the patient can look inside the imaging aperture for several minutes at a time without discomfort or tiredness. Patient should be instructed to look at the center of the green target, and not at the moving lights of the scan beam. (Figure 1).

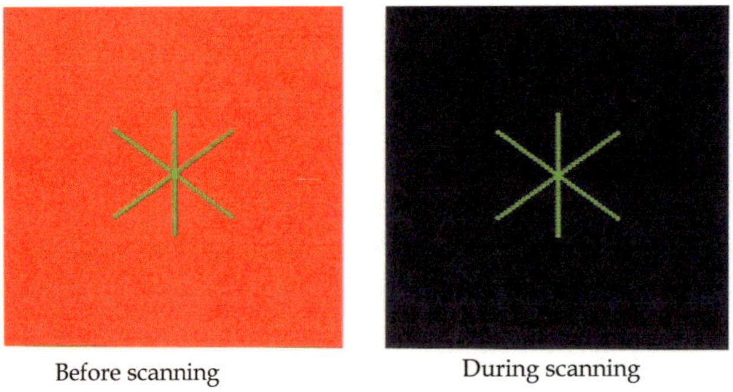

Figure 1. Pattern of targets seen by the patient during OCT procedure.

http://dx.doi.org/10.5772/53961

Anterior segment OCT uses light source with longer infrared wavelengths (1310 nm) to improve the penetration through light scattering tissues, such as sclera and limbus. Unlike posterior segment OCT, AS-OCT requires greater depth of field. AS-OCT also requires higher energy levels than retinal OCT systems. Visualization of retroiridial structures is limited in current AS-OCT, especially in presence of ocular surface opacities and heavy iris pigmentation (Goldsmith et al., 2005]. Currently Cirrus HD-OCT versions 4.0 and 5.0 cannot be used for anterior segment structures, however, one of the latest software updates of Stratus OCT (version 6.0) can measure corneal thickness and visualize structures of the anterior chamber angle.

UHR-OCT uses broadband light sources and has an axial resolution below 5 microns in the tissue.

Intraoperative 3D SD-OCT is the current hot spot in ophthalmology. These systems are separate from the operating microscope and surgery has to be halted while performing the scans. An ideal intraoperative OCT system must be integrated into the operating microscope with a head-up display so that real-time imaging of the operative field can be made without disrupting the surgery (Tang et al., 2010).

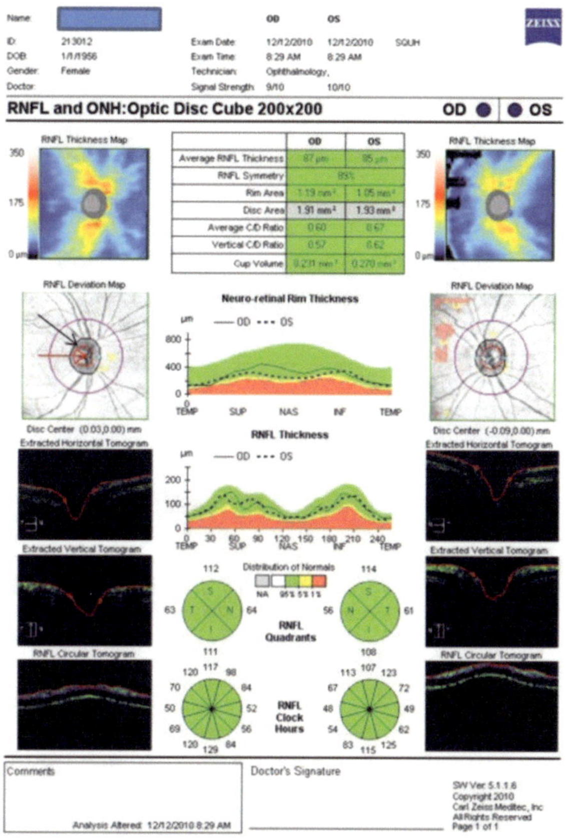

Figure 2. Optic disc cube in a normal patient. See text for details.

2.1. The optic disc cube (Figure 2)

This scan measures the retinal nerve fiber layer (RNFL) thickness in a 6 x 6-mm^2 area consisting of 200 x200 pixels (axial scans). The RNFL thickness is measured at each pixel and a RNFL thickness map is generated. The optic disc (black arrow) and the cup (red arrow) are represented in the center of the scan. A calculation circle of 3.46-mm diameter consisting of 256-A scans is automatically positioned around the optic disc. It is ideal to have signal strength ≥ 6 for the scans. The scan gives an hour-pattern, quadrant-pattern and mean RNFL thickness, which are color coded (white-thickest; green-normal; yellow-borderline, and red-abnormally thin). The printout gives all credible measurements about the RNFL thickness, rim area, disc area, cup-disc ratio and RNFL symmetry.

The scans of two eyes can be compared for symmetry. Latest models can detect saccadic eye movements with the line-scanning ophthalmoscope overlaid with OCT en face during the scanning. Images with motion artifact are rescanned. The SD-OCT has given a precise correlation between optic disc neuroanatomy and histomorphometric reconstruction, which in turn helps understand the pathogenesis in glaucoma (Alexandre et al., 2012; Strouthidis et al., 2009).

2.2. The macular cube (Figure 3)

Generates a cube of data through a 6mm square grid by acquiring a series of 28 horizontal scan lines each composed of 512 A-scans, except for the central vertical and horizontal scans, which are composed of 1024 A-scans each. There are two versions of the macular cube, 512x128 (Figure 3) and 200x200.

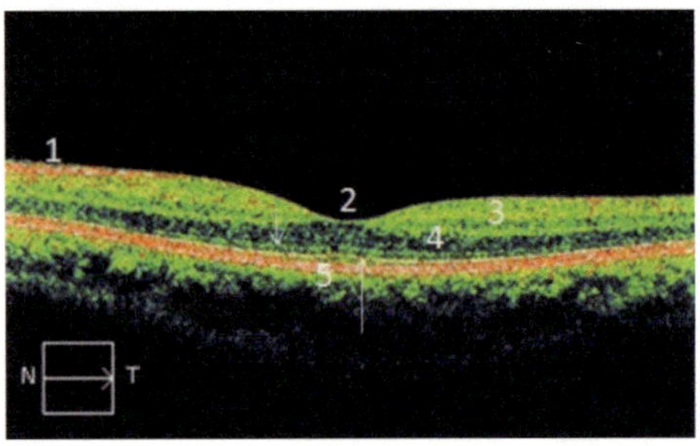

Figure 3. Macular Cube 512x128 in a normal patient. N-Nasal (left hand side of image); T-temporal (right hand side of image). 1-RNFL; 2- Normal foveal depression; 3- plexiform layer (orange-green); 4-Nuclear layer (black); 5-Retinal pigment epithelium (red band of high reflectivity); Short white arrow- External limiting membrane; long white arrow- junction of inner and outer segments of photoreceptors (area of high reflectivity)

The 512 x 128 module has greater resolution in each line from left to right but less resolution from top to bottom. The 200x200 module also has 6mm square grid and acquires 200 horizontal scans each composed of 200 A- scans, except for the central vertical and horizontal scans, which are composed of 1000 A-scans each. Detailed description of the basics of OCT and its images are available on line (Wali & Kharousi., 2012) A 3-D option offers an added advantage in defining the lesions (Figure 4).

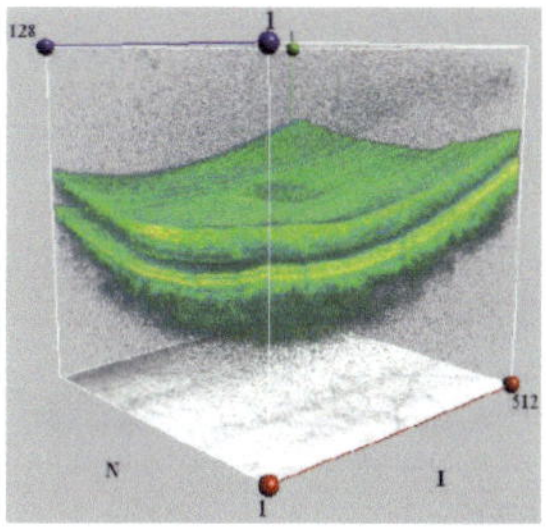

Figure 4. A look-alike of a 3-dimensional figure (here on a 2 dimension surface)

2.3. Anterior segment OCT

This is a custom-built, high speed ultra high resolution device which uses a 3-module superluminescent diode light source allowing an axial resolution of 2 to 3μm. This enables morphologic visualization of conjunctival and corneal architecture. (Shousa et al., 2011 & 2010). The noninvasive nature and quick acquisition time (seconds) makes AS-OCT an ideal imaging technique in handicapped and elderly patients.

3. Current applications of OCT in clinical ophthalmology

Optical coherence tomography provides both qualitative and quantitative (thickness and volume) analyses of the tissues examined in-situ. OCT has been exploited in evaluating both anterior and posterior segments of the eye.

The highest impact of OCT has been in aiding the diagnosis and following the response to treatment and in patients suffering from diabetic retinopathy (DR) (Cruz-Villegas et al., 2004), age-related macular degeneration (ARMD) (Mavro frides et al., 2004) and venous occlusions.

Other applications include imaging morphology and lesions of posterior hyaloid like vitreomacular traction (Figure 5), vitreomacular adhesion (Figure 6) (Kang et al., 2004), detection of fluid within and under the retina which may not be visible clinically. The retinal edema can be measured and localized to different retinal layers. Macular holes (Mavrofrides et al., 2005) and pseudoholes can be more accurately graded, defined and differentiated. Other indications include diagnosis and defining of epiretinal membranes (ERMs) (Mori et al., 2004), retinoschisis (Eriksson et al., 2004), retinal detachment, drug toxicities, RNFL thickness and optic disc parameters.

OCT should not be the only criteria for diagnosis of any ocular disease. Valid perspectives of patient's systemic and ocular disease, clinical examination, fluorescein angiography (FA), indocyanine green angiography (ICGA), biomicroscopy, and above all, the relevant history of the disease process should always be made partner with OCT imaging.

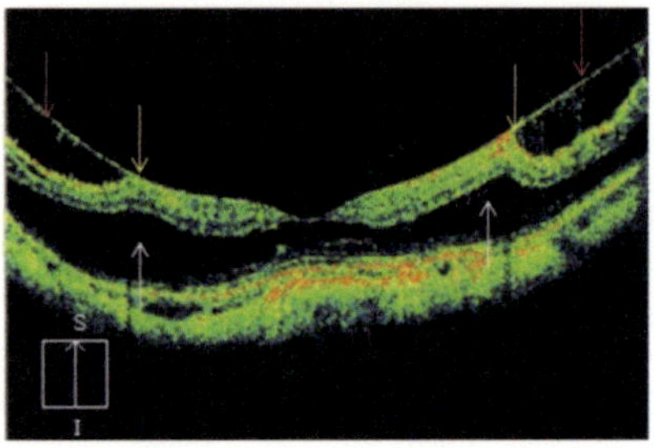

Figure 5. Vitreomacular traction (yellow arrows) by posterior hyaloid membrane (red arrows) causing retinoschisis (white arrows). S-superior (right side of image); I-Inferior (left side of image).

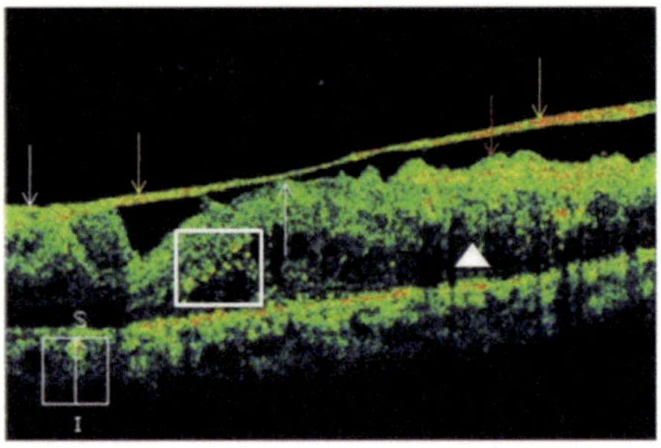

Figure 6. Vitreomacular adhesion: A taught thick posteior hyaloid face (yellow arrows) makes areas of adhesions (white arrow) with the retinal surface producing marked irregularity (bumps) of the retinal tissue (red arrow). Note the hard exudates (white box) and marked retinal thickening due to subretinal fluid (white triangle)

3.1. Anterior segment

There are several advantages of AS-OCT over conventional imaging methods like slit illumination, slit-scanning tomography, Scheimpflug imaging and ultrasound biomicroscopy (UBM). The imaging resolution of AS-OCT is higher than these modalities and gives high resolution cross-sectional 3D images of the anterior segment (Dawczynski et al., 2007; Tan et al., 2011; Goldsmith et al., 2005) Recent models of AS-OCT provide topographic analysis, anterior and posterior elevation maps of the cornea and reliable pachymetric maps (Milla et al., 2011; Nakagawa et al., 2011). It is an ideal research tool to demonstrate ciliary body contraction and lens movement during accommodation (Baikoff et al., 2004).

3.1.1. Cornea and refractive surgery

AS-OCT can be used to determine presurgical parameters in planning different anterior segment procedures. These parameters include anterior chamber depth, crystalline lens rise (distance between anterior pole of crystalline lens and the line joining two iridocorneal angle lines) and anterior chamber angle morphology with reference to the scleral spur (Dawczynski et al., 2007; Tan et al., 2011; Goldsmith et al., 2005). Such parameters can also be used to analyze postsurgical chamber angle dynamics and in intraocular lens (IOL) power calculations (Dinc et al.,

2010; Tan et al., 2011) Phakic IOL is becoming a very popular refractive surgery technique for treatment of high refractive errors. AS-OCT simulates the position of the phakic IOL before surgery by evaluation of anterior segment structures (Mamalis N., 2010). Postoperatively AS-OCT can visualize the contact between the collamer refractive lens and the crystalline lens (Lindland et al., 2010). In cataract surgery AS-OCT has been instrumental in analyzing the structure, integrity and configuration of corneal incisions after cataract surgery (Jagow Von & Kohnen., 2009) yielding information about corneal wound architecture, Descemet's detachment and wound leaks. Studies with AS-OCT have also revealed that corneal epithelial closure after cataract surgery was completed in 1-8 days (Can et al., 2011; Torres et al., 2006), postoperative Descemet's detachment occurred in 40-82% of patients on day one (Fukuda et al., 2011] and that stromal hydration persisted for up to 7 days.

AS-OCT has proved very useful in early recognition of localized or total graft dislocation in Descemet stripping automated endothelial keratoplasty (DSAEK), especially in eyes with corneal edema and limited anterior chamber visualization (Kymionis et al., 2010). The technique can also aid in diagnosis of eccentric trephination and inverse implantation of the donor (Ide et al., 2008; Kymionis et al., 2007; Suh et al., 2008). AS-OCT has been pivotal in documenting the cause of hyperopic shift in DSAEK eyes, which was induced by a high ratio of central graft thickness to peripheral graft thickness (Yoo et al., 2008). Epithelial in growth in refractive surgery can be confirmed by OCT images (Stahl et al., 2007).

OCT imaging and femtosecond laser-assisted surgeries are the most rapidly advancing technologies in modern day ophthalmology. Thickness is an important parameter in refractive surgery and no technique other than OCT can give accurate, uniform and predictable thickness measurements before, during and after surgery. The pachymetry map of AS-OCT can be used in femtosecond laser-assisted astigmatic keratotomy, LASIK enhancement and intrastromal tunnel preparation for intracorneal ring segments (Hoffart et al., 2009; Nubile et al., 2009). AS-OCT is very helpful in determining the accurate depth of the arcuate incisions, and in the postoperative follow up of patient with femtosecond astigmatic keratotomy and intracorneal ring segments. The images can explain the reasons behind unexpected postsurgical surprises (Yoo & Hurmeric., 2011). Femtosecond-assisted lamellar keratoplasty (FALK) is a highly promising refractive surgical technique that requires OCT data in accurate presurgical planning (Yoo et al., 2008). These procedures include anterior lamellar keratoplasty and deep anterior lamellar keratoplasty. AS-OCT imaging is the first step to measure the depth of anterior stromal scar and this determines the preparation of the donor and the recipient corneas. The morphology of the perfect match (donor and recipient) is confirmed by AS-OCT imaging. AS-OCT helps in careful planning of structure, thickness and shape of LASIK flap (Li et al., 2007; Rosas et al., 2011]. It is the depth of corneal incisions as obtained from AS-OCT that determines the success of new surgical techniques like femtosecond-assisted corneal biopsies, corneal tattooing and collagen crosslinking (Kymionis et al., 2009; Kanellopoulos et al.,2009; Nagy et al., 2009).

New platforms provide integrated OCT systems in the operating microscopes to perform the anterior segment procedures like corneal incisions, continuous curvilinear capsulorrhexis, nucleus softening, lens fragmentation, and focusing the laser in 3D manner in femtosecond-assisted cataract surgery (William et al., 2011; Wang et al., 2009).

Another milestone in OCT technology has been development of intraoperative 3D SD-OCT in the supine position (Dayani et al., 2009). This technique has been used for intraoperative evaluation of the presence of interface fluid between the donor and the recipient corneas in DSAEK.

3.1.2. Ocular surface disorders

OCT can be used for assessment of conjunctival and corneal tissue planes with high axial resolution. (Christopoulas et al., 2007 ; Shousha et al., 2011]. The technique acts as an adjuvant tool in diagnosing ocular surface squamous neoplasia and pterygia (Jeremy et al.,2012). OCT is in potential use for diagnosis and patient follow-up during the course of medical treatment and continued watch for recurrence of neoplasia without any need for repeated biopsies. Also the technique may be helpful in determining the extent of the tumor to facilitate its complete excision. AS-OCT guided subtenon injections of drugs like triamcinolone has reduced chances of inadvertent perforations and unwanted targets.

3.1.3. Glaucoma (anterior segment)

Recently Fourier-domain OCT has been used to examine the position, patency and the interior entrance site of the anterior chamber aqueous tube shunts. This high resolution OCT shows exact position of the AC entrance relative to Schwalbe's line and growth of fibrous tissue between the tube and the corneal endothelium. Such findings could not be seen with slit-lamp examination or lower resolution time-domain OCT. The tube position visualized by slitlamp examination differed from OCT finding (Jiang et al., 2012). OCT is also very helpful in correlating the clinical and visual field changes in glaucoma and ocular hypertension patients (Figure 7 & 8).

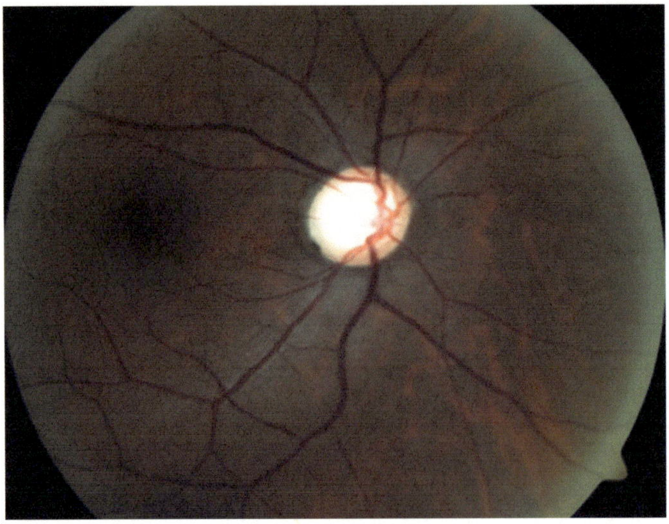

Figure 7. Fundus photo showing glaucomatous cupping temporaly.

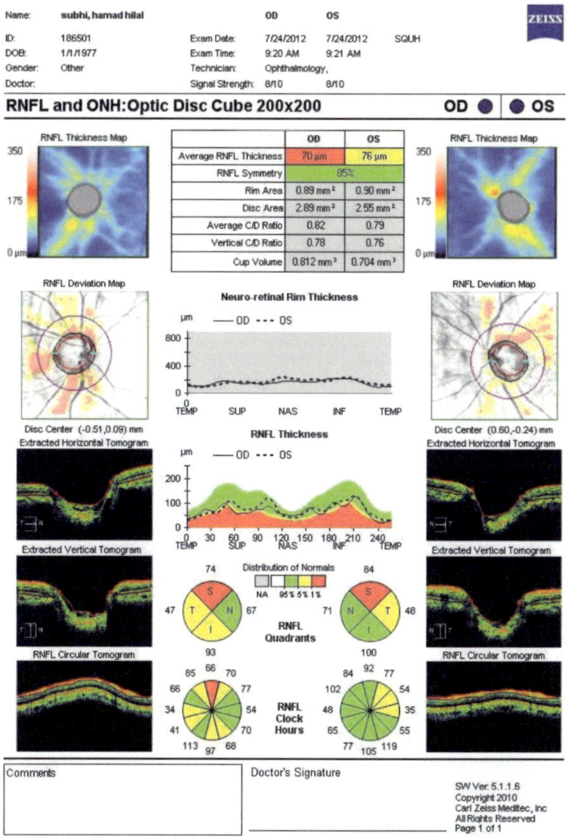

Figure 8. OCT printout of optic disc cube showing glaucomatous changes. The red measurements indicate abnormal thinning of RNFL, yellow areas represent borderline thickness of RNFL and green areas mean normal thickness of RNFL.

3.1.4. Ultrahigh Resolution (UHR) OCT

Ultrahigh resolution (UHR) OCT has been more practical and advantageous over confocal microscopy in making a clear distinction between morphologic and histopathologic features between normal and abnormal epithelium in ocular surface squamous neoplasia and pterygia. This is so because OCT is a noncontact method, has rapid image capture, and provides a cross-sectional view of the tissue. One of the recent clinical applications of UHR- OCT is the identification of the opaque bubble layer as a bright white area in mid stroma in femtosecond laser-assisted LASIK flap creation (Nordan et al., 2003). This technique has been of immense help to refractive surgeons in analyzing the flap integrity, indistinct flap interface or epithelial breakthrough in LASIK surgery (Seider et al., 2008; Ide et al., 2009; Ide et al., 2010). OCT is not a substitute for histopathologic specimens; however, it can be a potential noninvasive diagnostic adjuvant in diagnosis and surveillance of anterior segment pathologies of the eye.

3.2. Posterior segment

OCT now has a role in varied types of posterior segment pathologies (inflammatory, non-inflammatory, degenerative, vascular, traumatic, neoplastic, and metastatic) where the technique clearly defines the levels of various pathologic lesions in the posterior hyaloid, retina, retinal pigment epithelium and choroid, which in turn defines the mode and success of therapy. Such lesions may be superficial (epiretinal and vitreous membranes (Figures 6, 9 and 10), cotton wool spots, retinal hemorrhages, hard exudates (Figure 11), cysts (Figure 12), retinal fibrosis, and retinal scars (Figure 13) or deep (drusen-Figure 14), retinal pigment epithelial hyperplasia and detachment (Figure 15), intraretinal and subretinal neovascular membranes (Figure 16), scarring (figure 13) and pigmented lesions).

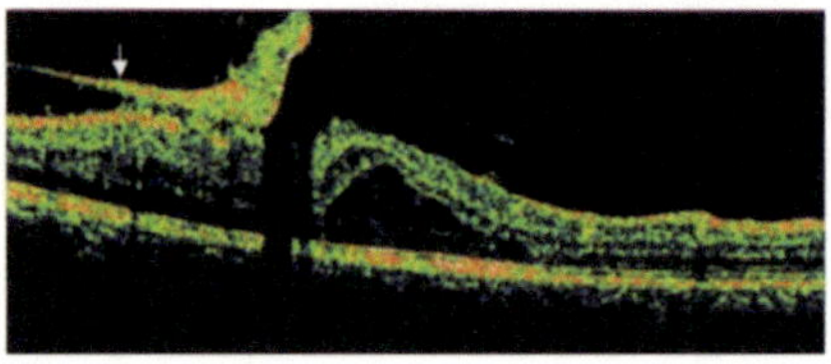

Figure 9. Epiretinal membrane (arrow) causing ripping of retinal tissue

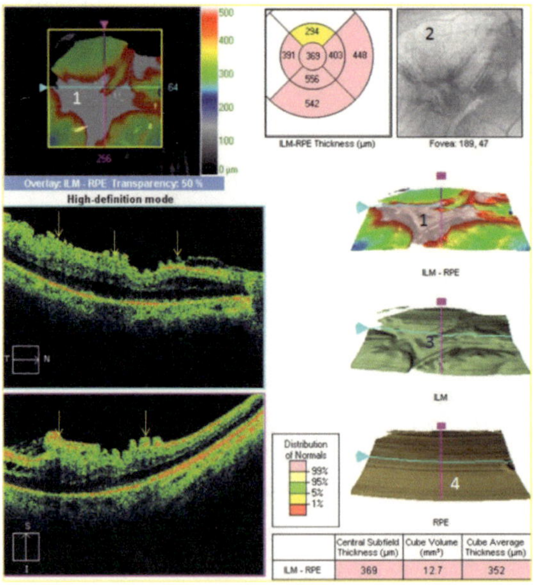

Figure 10. Retinal infoldings due to epiretinal membrane: 1: color map showing marked thickening (silver white and red areas) of ILM (internal limiting membrane)-RPE (retinal pigment epithelium) interface. 2: grey tone video image showing irregular surface with striations due to fibrous membrane. 3: ILM map showing marked irregularity due to contraction of the fibrous membrane. 4: A relatively intact RPE. Note the teeth-like infoldings of the retinal surface (yellow arrows) produced by ERM.

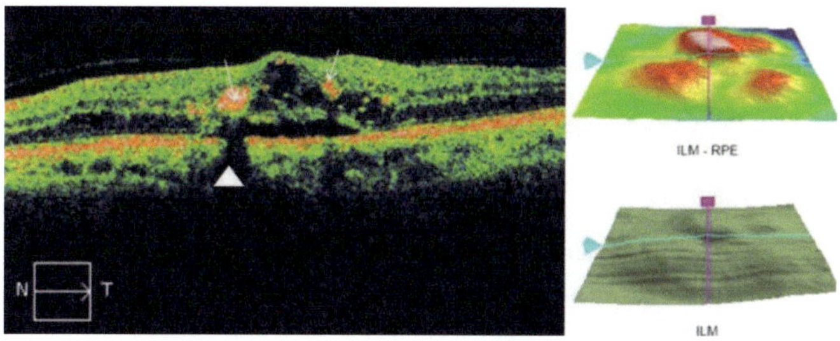

Figure 11. Hard exudates (white arrows). White triangle indicates the shadow cast by the exudate. The ILM-RPE color map shows three humps due to exudates.

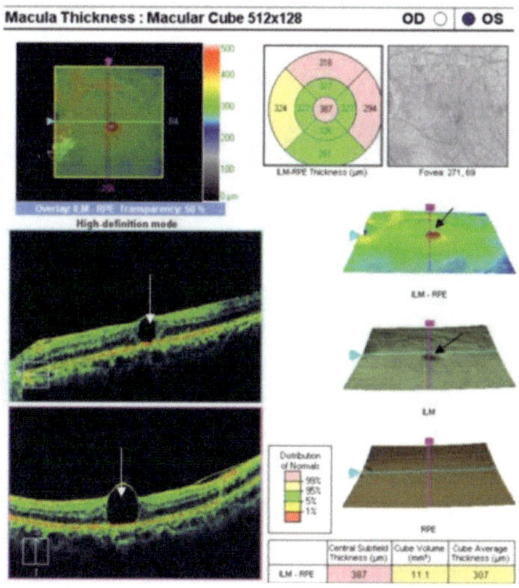

Figure 12. Solitary macular cyst (arrows). Note the blisters (black arrows) in the color map, corresponding to the cyst.

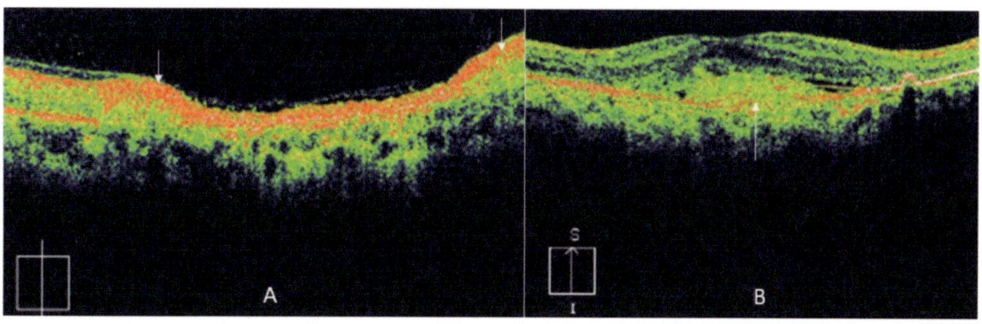

Figure 13. A: Extensive retinal scarring in a thin atrophic retina (orange red hyperreflective band between arrows). 13B- Scarring following involution of CNVM (arrow)

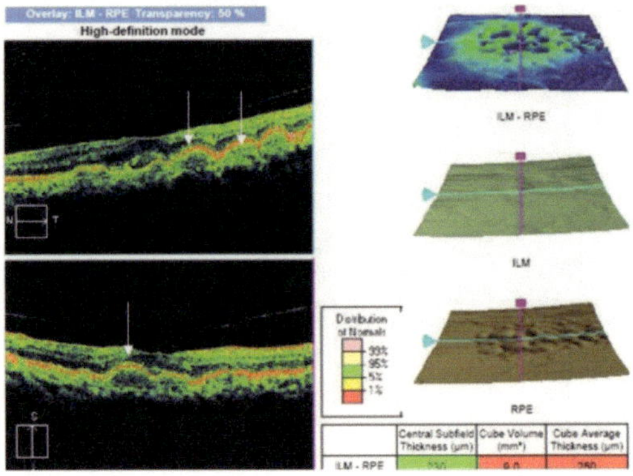

Figure 14. Drusen with bumps in the RPE (arrows). The drusen bumps produce characteristic humps in the color maps of ILM-RPE interface.

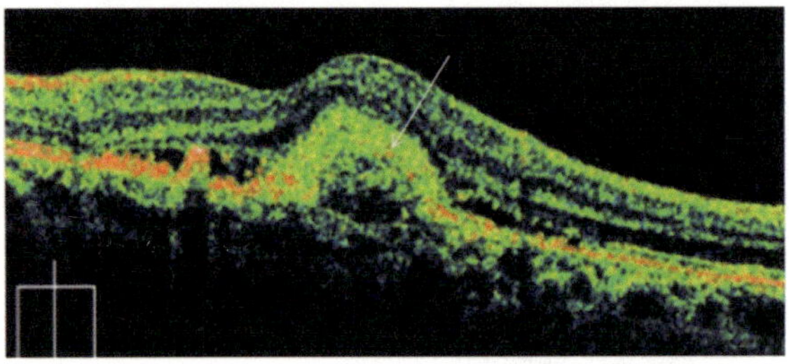

Figure 15. Thickened, irregular and detached RPE (arrow)

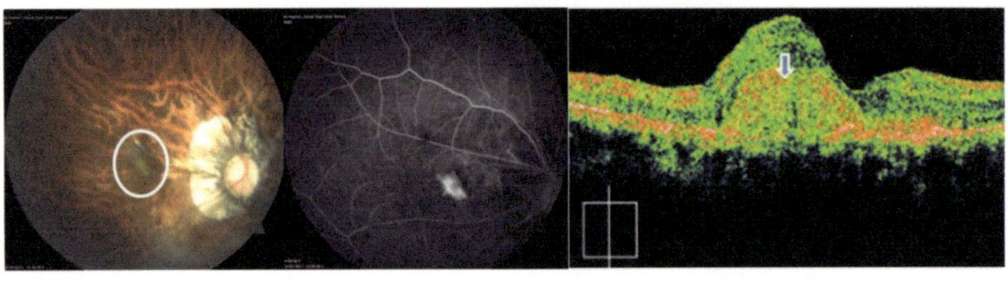

Figure 16. Myopic CNVM: Fundus photo gives a vivid description of myopic peripapillary atropy and a greyish white neovascular membrane in the macular area (encircled). FFA shows characteristic leakage corresponding to the area of neovascular membrane. OCT image depicts a hyperreflective subfoveal CNVM with increased retinal thickness (thick arrow).

3.2.1. Disorders of vitreous and posterior hyaloid

Vitreomacular traction (VMT) and vitreomacular adhesion (VMA) may be difficult to detect clinically. OCT is extremely helpful in such cases by showing hyperreflectivity. The traction by the membrane to the retina induces deformations of the retinal surface (Figure 17).

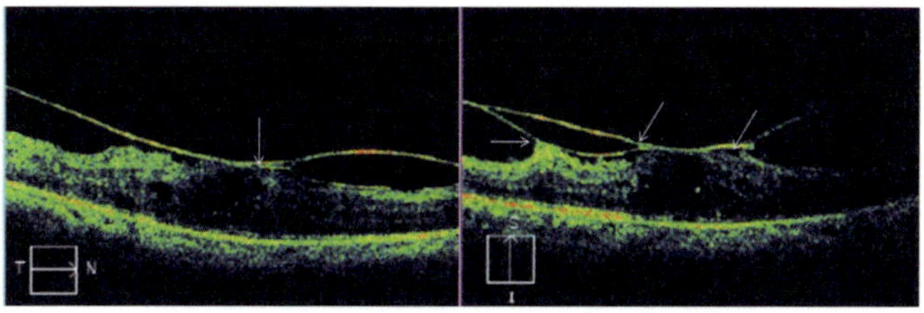

Figure 17. Vitreomacular traction. Note the multiple areas of traction caused by taught posterior hyaloid on retinal tissue (arrows).

3.2.2. Retinal edema

The most common primary cause of retinal thickening is edema. One of the major achievements of OCT has been quantitative assessment of retinal edema in terms of measuring its thickness and volume, evaluate the progression of the pathologic process, and monitor surgical or non-surgical intervention (Kang et al., 2004). Retinal edema may manifest in different categories:

Focal or diffuse edema: Common causes include diabetic retinopathy, central retinal venous occlusion, branch retinal venous occlusion, arterial occlusion, hypertensive retinopathy, preeclampsia, eclampsia, uveitis, retinitis pigmentosa and retraction of internal limiting membrane. OCT helps in diagnosis of edema in preclinical stage when there may be no or few visible changes.

Cystoid macular edema (CME): (Figure 18) Common causes of CME include diabetic retinopathy, age-related macular degeneration (ARMD), venous occlusions, pars planitis, Uveitis, pseudophakos, Irvine-Gass syndrome, Birdshot retinopathy and retinitis pigmentosa. OCT usually shows diffuse cystic spaces in the outer nuclear layer of central macula, and increased retinal thickness which is maximally concentric on the fovea (Mavrofrides et al., 2004).

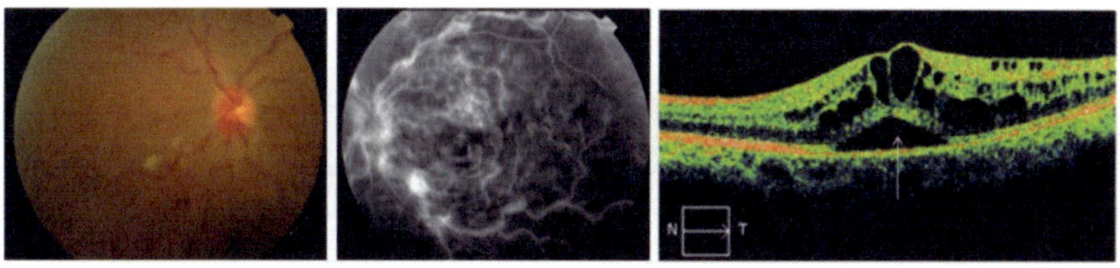

Figure 18. Cystoid macular edema in a patient with CRVO. Color fundus image shows disc hemorrhage, venous tortuosity, cotton wool exudates and retinal hemorrhages. FFA shows characteristic venous staining, leakge and blocked fluorescence due to underlying hemorrhage. OCT image depicts marked increase in retinal thickness due to edema. Note the intraretinal cysts and subretinal fluid (arrow).

Serous retinal detachment: The cysts of retinal edema over a period of time loose their walls and merge together forming single or multiple pools of fluid within retinal layers or between retinal pigment epithelium (RPE) and the sensory retina (Villate et al., 2004.) (Figure 19)

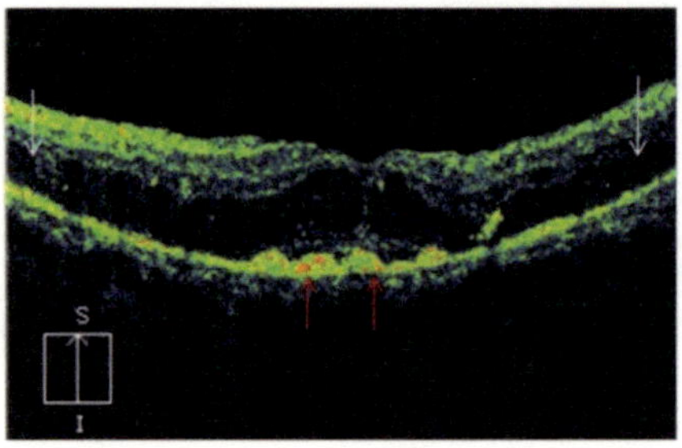

Figure 19. Serous retinal detachment (dark zone between white arrows) in a patient with severe nonproliferative diabetic retinopathy. Red arrows indicate subfoveal exudates.

3.2.3. Retinal pigment epithelial detachment (Figure 20)

Its pathophysiology involves passage of serous fluid from the choriocapillaries to the sub-RPE space or collection of blood under RPE causing its separation and elevation from the Bruch's membrane. OCT scans show a classical dome-shaped detachment of the RPE with intact contour in early stages (Figure 14).

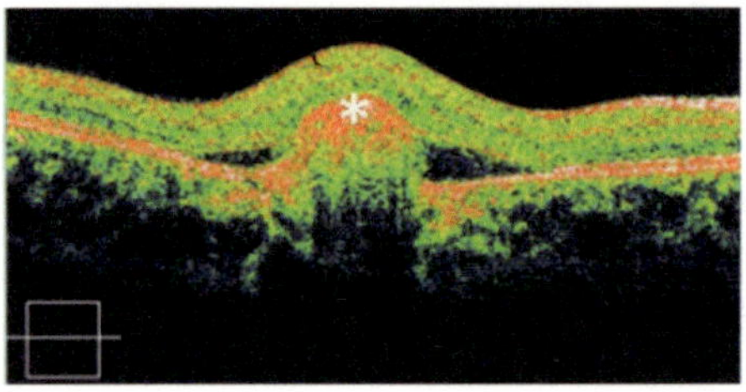

Figure 20. RPE detachment with hyperplasia (asterisk).

3.2.4. Epiretinal membranes (ERM)

Epiretinal membranes are fibroglial proliferations on the vitreo-retinal interface (Figure 10). They may be sequel of chronic intraocular inflammations, venous occlusions, trauma, post-surgical or may be idiopathic. OCT helps in confirming such membranes (Suzuki et al., 2003; Massin et al., 2000).

3.2.5. Secondary retinal lesions

OCT is important to document the presence, degree and extent of subretinal fluid (Villate et al., 2004), assessment of the level of retinal infiltrates and detect macular edema in patients with chronic uveitis where hazy media may prevent clinical examination to find the cause of reduced vision (Antcliff et al., 2002; Markomichelakis et al., 2004).

3.2.6. Retinoschisis

It is the separation or splitting of the neurosensory retina into an inner (vitreous) and outer (choroidal) layer with severing of neurons and complete loss of visual function in the affected area (Figure 21). Typically the split is in the outer plexiform layer. In reticular retinoschisis, which is less common, splitting occurs at the level of nerve fiber layer. Retinoschisis may be degenerative, myopic, juvenile or idiopathic. Presence of vitreoretinal traction is an important cause. OCT reveals wide space with vertical palisades and splitting of the retina into a thinner outer layer and thicker inner layer (Eriksson et al., 2004).

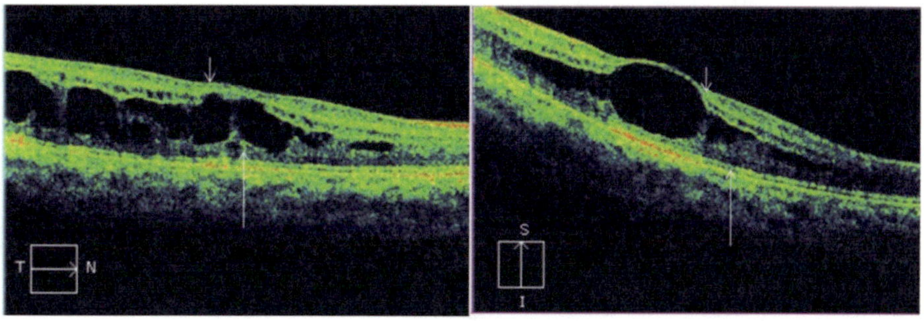

Figure 21. Retinoschisis: Note the splitting of retina into inner (small arrow) and outer layers (large arrow)

3.2.7. Macular holes

Lamellar hole: OCT depicts a homogenous increase in foveal and perifoveal retinal thickness, and presence of residual retinal tissue at the base of the hole (Figure 22).

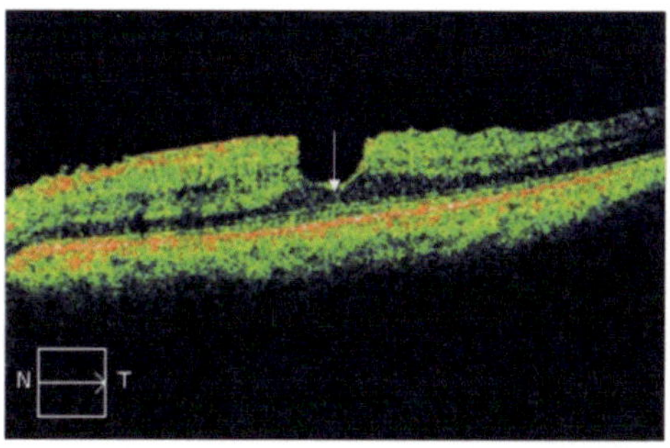

Figure 22. OCT image of a lamellar thickness macular hole with residual retinal tissue remaining between the base of the hole (arrow) and the RPE.

Full thickness macular hole: Majority of macular holes are idiopathic. Other causes include trauma, high myopia, vascular lesions (DR, venous occlusions, and hypertensive retinopathy) and subretinal neovascularization. OCT features in a full thickness macular hole include complete absence of foveal retinal reflectivity with no residual retinal tissue. Thickened retinal margins around the hole with reduced intraretinal reflectivity are clearly seen in such cases (Figure 23).

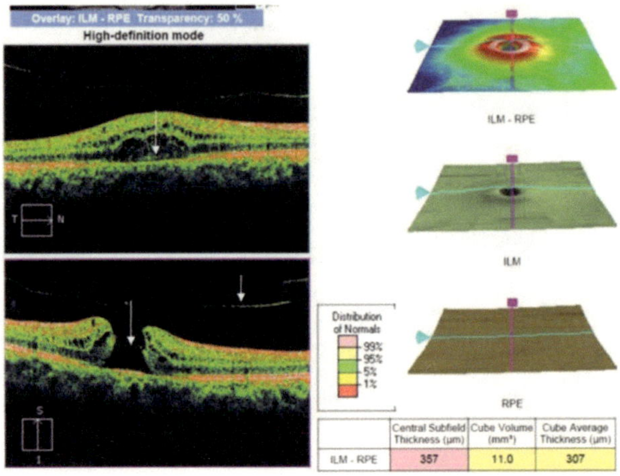

Figure 23. OCT (S-1): A full thickness macular hole (long arrow) in a diabetic patient with detached posterior hyaloid (short arrow). The T-N axis shows subretinal fluid collection (arrow). Color map: Top: red circle delineates edema; Middle: delineates a hole with elevated margins; Bottom: normal RPE.

3.2.8. Diabetic retinopathy

OCT is a vital tool in the hands of a vitreoretinal surgeon that aids in diagnosis, treatment and follow up of patients with DR. (Cruz-Villegas et al., 2004; Schaudig et al., 2000).

OCT features in DR include retinal edema, cotton wool spots, exudates, hemorrhages and ischemia. (Figures 24, 25)

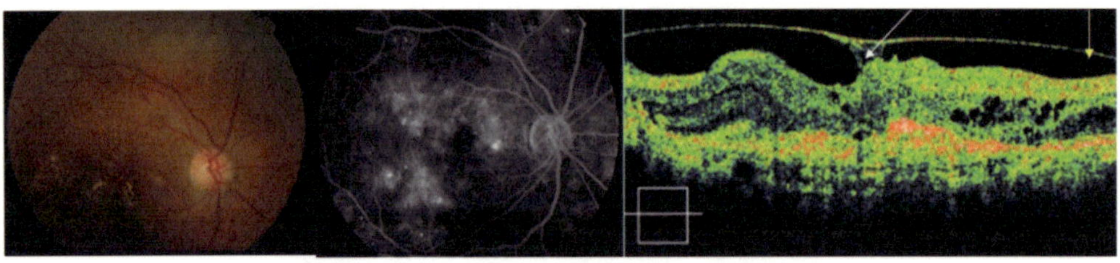

Figure 24. NPDR: color fundus photo shows classical moderate to severe NPDR with hemorrhages, exudates and maculopathy. FA shows retinal edema confined mainly to macular area. The foveal avascular zone is enlarged. OCT image shows VMA (white arrow), detached posterior hyaloid (yellow arrow), retinal thickening and intraretinal edema.

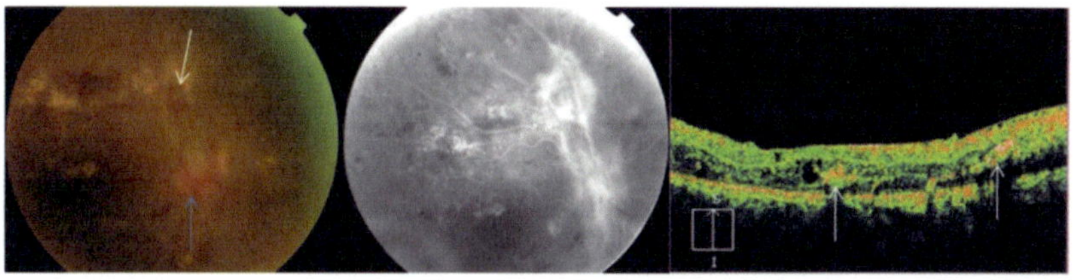

Figure 25. Proliferative diabetic retinopathy (PDR): Color fundus photo shows neovascularization of disc (NVD-blue arrow), neovascularization elsewhere (NVE- white arrow) and exudates. FFA shows corresponding leakge of dye. OCT image shows exudates (white arrows), a thin ERM and mild retinal edema.

3.2.9. Drug toxicities

OCT studies have started evaluating the retinal / macular toxic side effects of systemic drugs like hydroxychloroquine (Marmor., 2012), chloroquine (Korah and Kuriakose., 2008), tamoxifen (Hager et al., 2010), ethambutol (Menon et al., 2009), vigabatrin (Moseng et al., 2011) and tadalafil. (Coscas et al., 2012) Besides, the technique is being used in many research centers for studying retinal effects of a varied number of compounds in animal models.

3.2.10. Inflammatory lesions

OCT displays common associations of inflammation like edema, hemorrhage and scarring (Figure 26).

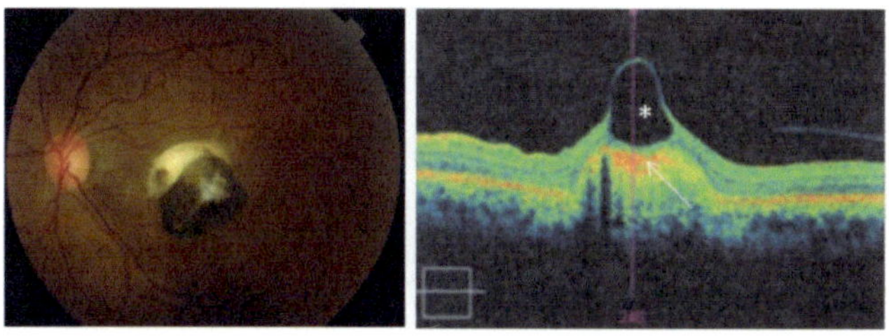

Figure 26. Color fundus image of a healed lesion of macular toxoplasmosis. OCT image shows scarring (arrow) associated with a retinal cyst (asterix).

3.2.11. Trauma and foreign bodies

Though clinical details of retinal foreign bodies may be quite discernible superficially, OCT gives a detailed description of the retinal layers affected and the sequel of impacted deeper foreign bodies (Figure 27). The sequel of blunt eye injuries may be sub-clinical and OCT helps in determining the cause of unexplained reduced vision in such cases (Figure 27A).

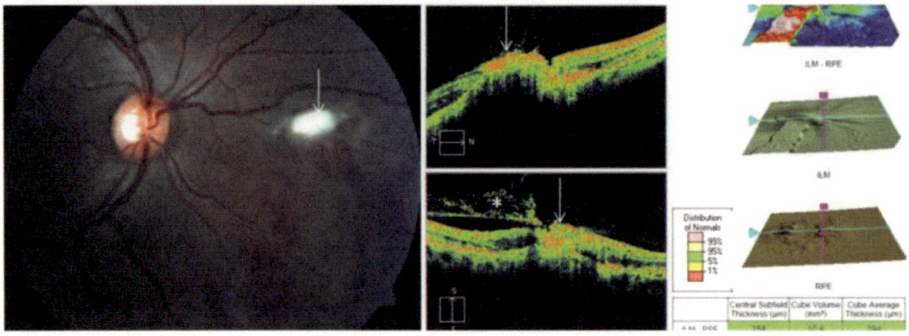

Figure 27. Embedded metallic retinal foreign body (arrow) with inferior retinal hemorrhage. OCT image showing retinal deformation with fibrosis (arrow) and vitreo-retinal debri (asterix). Note the deformation of the ILM-RPE color maps caused by fibrosis.

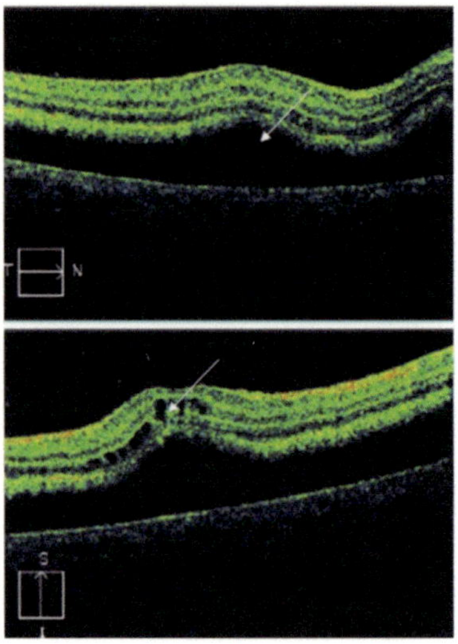

Figure 28. A(adobe): Submacular retinal detachment (arrows) in a 17 year old boy who sustained blunt eye injury after being hit by a football in the eye.

3.2.12. Neoplastic /metastatic lesions

OCT yields valuable information in such lesions especially when clinical examination may not be decisive due to media opacities (Figure 29).

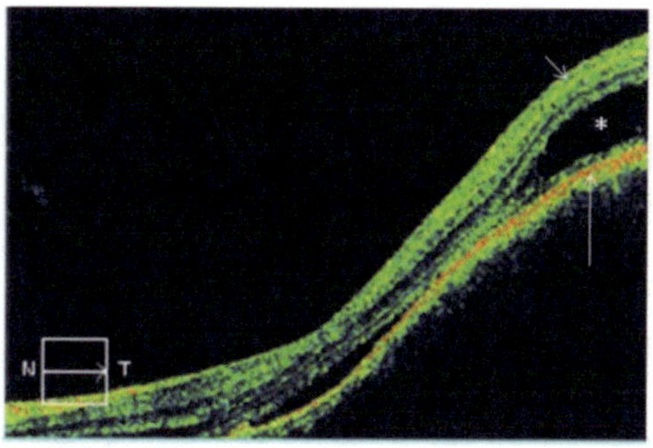

Figure 29. A 57 year old male with metastatic subretinal lesion. OCT image shows large dome shaped retinal (short arrow) and retinal pigment epithelium (long arrow) detachment associated with subretinal fluid (asterix).

The most exploited use of OCT has been in the field of treatment guidelines and response to therapies in diabetic retinopathy (figure 30), retinal vascular occlusions (figure 31), vascular lesions (figure 32), age related macular degeneration (figure 33), and intraocular inflammations. Physicians, who are used to OCT technology, feel more confident in diagnosing and managing such retinal disorders.

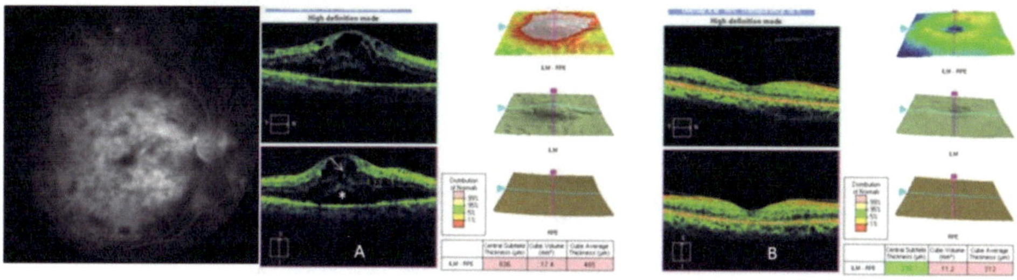

Figure 30. Diabetic macular edema: FFA shows diffuse leakage of dye in the macular area. OCT image (A): before treatment: diffuse macular edema with cystoid spaces (arrow) and subretinal fluid (asterix; central subfoveal thickness 836 microns). The septa (arrow) between retinal cysts are comprised of Müller's fibers. OCT image (B): dramatic improvement in retinal edema (central subfoveal thickness 230 microns) after intravitreal bevacizumab injections.

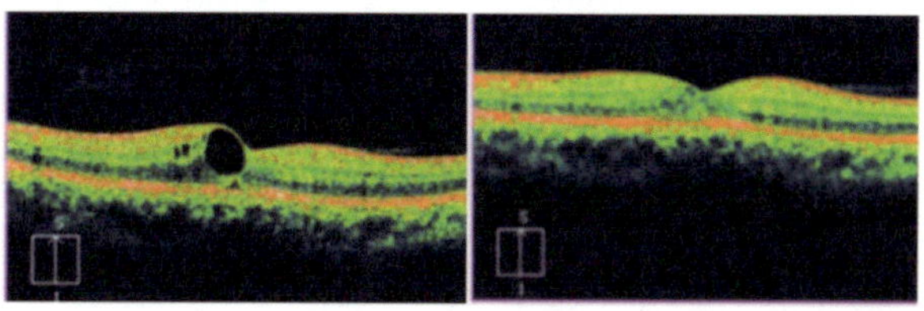

Figure 31. Left: Cystoid macular edema in a patient with branch retinal vein occlusion before therapy. Right: Two months after two intravitreal injections of bevacizumab the edema had resolved and normal foveal architecture was restored.

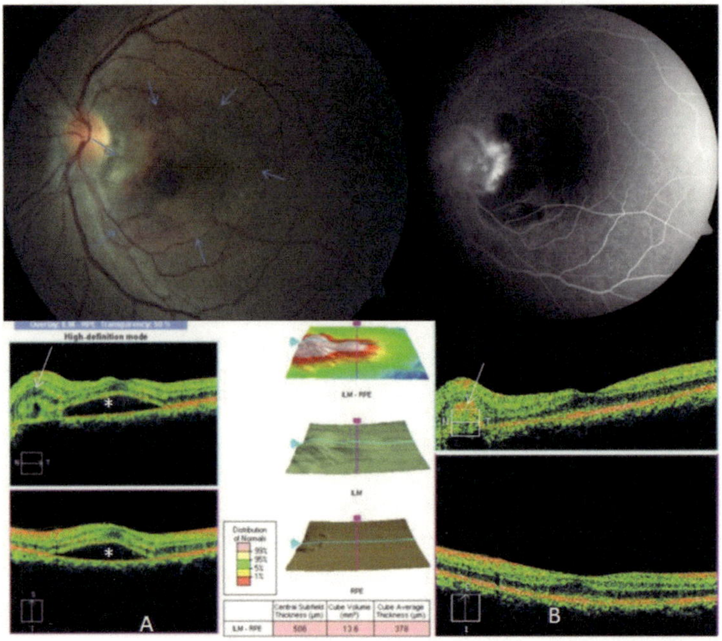

Figure 32. Juxtapapillary choroidal neovascular membrane in a 39 year old male. Color fundus photo shows the hemorrhage in deeper retinal layers with a circumscribed area of subretinal exudation (delineated by blue arrows). FFA shows leakge of dye from the juxtapapillary neovascular membrane. The dark area corresponds to blocked fluorescence due to hemorrhage. OCT image (A-before treatment) shows classical CNVM mound (arrow) with subretinal fluid in supero-temporal quadrant (asterix). OCT image (B) 18 weeks after three intravitreal injections of anti-VEGF drug ranibizumab shows brick-red organization (fibrosis) of CNVM (arrow) and resolution of subretinal fluid.

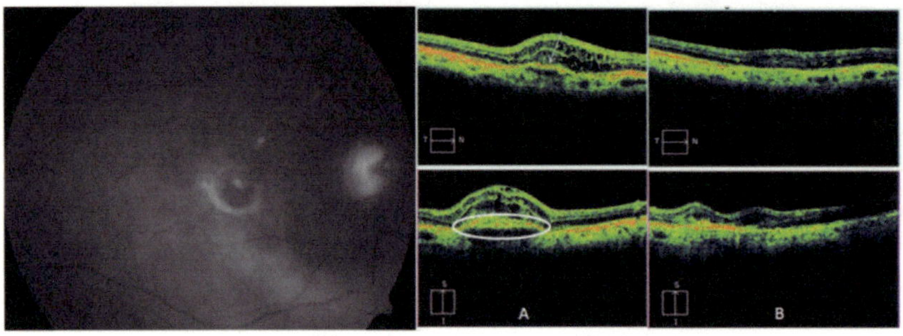

Figure 33. Age-related macular degeneration with CNVM. FFA shows a ring and central spot of hyperfluorescence in the macular area. OCT image A (30 April 2012) shows active CNVM (ovoid) with retinal edema and RPE deformity (arrow). The patient received two injections of intravitreal anti-VEGF drug ranibizumab. OCT image B (30 May 2012) shows marked regression of CNVM and retinal edema although retinal contour is altered.

Other therapeutic applications of OCT include accurate assessment of outcome of the effect of pharmacological or surgical interventions like photodynamic therapy (PDT), transpupillary thermotherapy, vitreoretinal surgery, anti-VEGF therapy, intravitreal steroid therapy and therapeutic Intravitreal implants (Rogers et al., 2002).

Recently OCT has confirmed benefit of intravitreal recombinant truncated human plasma serine protease ocriplasmin in treatment of non-symptomatic vitreomacular adhesion including macular hole (Decroos et al., 2012; Stalmans et al., 2010). OCT stays as sheet anchor in confirmation of successful surgical closure of macular holes (Jumper et al., 2000; Sato et al., 2003). In partial or unsuccessful surgeries, OCT evaluates the retinal anatomy to find reason for poor visual outcome.

4. Pediatric ophthalmology

SD-OCT allows detection of subclinical anatomic changes in neonates and infants, although experience on its use in retinopathy of prematurity (ROP) is limited (Chavala et al., 2009; Vinekar et al., 2010; Muni et al., 2010; Maldonado et al., 2010; Lee et al., 2011). Cystoid macular edema (CME) can be detected by SD-OCT in premature infants at risk for ROP but not when using indirect ophthalmoscopy (Maldonado et al., 2011). SD-OCT could be useful in detecting CME in neonates with mild and advanced ROP (Vinekar et al., 2011). Tomographic thickness measurements of cystoid macular edema in ROP predict the risk of requiring laser treatment or developing plus disease or ROP stage 3 (Maldonado et al., 2012). OCT is proving innovative in studying the macular characteristics in amblyopic eyes where the average thickness of foveolar neuroretina has been found to be larger than that of normal eyes (Wang et al., 2012)

5. Limitations of OCT

As with any new technology, limitations are inherent and so are with UHR-OCT. In anterior segment, leukoplakic or hyperreflective lesions often cast shadows on the underlying tissue. This may hide the diagnosis of underlying pathology.

6. Future strategies in OCT

Besides having OCT integrated slit lamp, increasing scanning speed and better axial resolution which would allow us to visualize tissues at the cellular level would be and should be the objective of future OCT imaging.

Author details

Nadia Al Kharousi, Upender K. Wali and Sitara Azeem

Department of Ophthalmology, College of Medicine and Health Sciences, Sultan Qaboos University, Muscat, Oman

References

[1] Huang D, Swanson EA, Lin CP, Schuman JS, Stinson WG, et al. (1991). Optical coherence tomography. Science, Vol. 254, No. 5035, (Nov), pp.1178-1181.

[2] Hrynchak P, Simpson T. (2007). Optical coherence tomography: an introduction to the technique and its use. Optom Vis Sci, Vol. 77, No. 7, (Jul), pp. 347-356.

[3] Ryan SJ. Retina, 4th edn, vol. 2. Elsevier Mosby 2006:1533-1556.

[4] Leung CK, Cheung CY, Weinreb RN, et al. (2009). Retinal nerve fiber layer imaging with spectral –domain optical coherence tomography: a variability and diagnostic performance study. Ophthalmology, Vol. 116, No. 7, (July), pp. 1257-63.

[5] Leung CK, Chiu V, Weinreb RN, et al. (2011). Evaluation of retinal nerve fiber layer progression in glaucoma: a comparison between spectral –domain and time – domain optical coherence tomography. Ophthalmology, Vol. 118, No.8, (Aug), pp. 1558 -62.

[6] Wang J, Conway TM, Yuan Y, Shen M, Cui L. (2010). Tear meniscus volume measured with ultra-high resolution OCT in dry eye after restasis treatment. ARVO Meeting Abstracts, 51 (Abstract 6266).

[7] Shen M, Wang MR, Yuan Y et al. (2010). SD-OCT with prolonged scan depth for imaging the anterior segment of the eye. Ophthal. Surg. Lasers Imaging, Vol. 41, No. 6, pp. S65–S69.

[8] Shousha MA, Perez VL, Wang J et al. (2010). Use of ultra-high-resolution optical coherence tomography to detect in vivo characteristics of Descemet's membrane in Fuchs' dystrophy. Ophthalmology, Vol. 117, No. 6, pp. 1220–1227.

[9] Goldsmith JA, Li Y, Chalita MR et al. (2005). Anterior chamber width measurement by high-speed optical coherence tomography Ophthalmology, Vol. 112, No. 2, pp. 238–244.

[10] Tang M, Chen A, Li Y, Huang D. (2010). Corneal power measurement with Fourier-domain optical coherence tomography. J. Cataract Refract. Surg., Vol. 36, No. 12, pp. 2115–2122.

[11] Alexandre SCR, Glen P. Sharpe, Hongli Yang, Marcelo TN, Claude FB, Balwantray CC. (2012). Optic Disc Margin Anatomy in Patients with Glaucoma and Normal Controls with Spectral Domain Optical Coherence Tomography. Ophthalmology Vol. 119, No.4, (Apr), pp. 738-747.

[12] Strouthidis NG, Yang H, Fortune B, et al. (2009). Detection of optic nerve head canal opening within histomorphometric and spectral domain optical coherence tomography data sets. Invest Ophthalmol Vis Sci, Vol. 50, No. 1, (Jan), pp. 214-23.

[13] Strouthidis NG, Yang H, Reynaud JF, et al. (2009). Comparison of clinical and spectral domain optical coherence tomography optic disc margin anatomy. Invest Ophthalmol Vis Sci, Vol. 50, No. 10, pp. 4709-18.

[14] Wali UK, Kharousi N. (2012). Selected Topics in Optical Coherence Tomography. In: Gangjun Liu, editor. Clinical Applications of Optical Coherence Tomography in Ophthalmology, Croatia; InTech publishing Inc; 2012, p 197-238.

[15] Shousha MA, Karp CL, Perez VL, et al. (2011). Diagnosis and management of conjunctival and corneal intraepithelial neoplasia using ultra high –resolution optical coherence tomography .Ophthalmology, Vol. 118,No. 8, pp. 1531 -7.

[16] Shousha MA, Perez VL, Wang J, et al. (2010). Use of ultra-high resolution Optical Coherence Tomography to detect in-vivo characteristics of Descemet's membrane in Fuch's dystrophy. Ophthalmology, Vol. 117, No.6, pp.1220-7.

[17] Cruz-Villegas V, Flynn HW Jr. (2004). Diabetic retinopathy. In: Schuman JS, Puliafito CA, Fujimoto JG, eds. Optical coherence tomography of ocular diseases. Thorofare, NJ: SLACK, Inc., 2004:157-214.

[18] Mavrofrides EC, Villate N, Rosenfeld PJ et al. [eds]. (2004). Optical coherence tomography of ocular diseases. In: Schuman JS, Puliafito CA, Fujimoto JG [eds]. Optical coherence tomography of ocular diseases. Thorofare, NJ: SLACK, Inc.; 2004:243-343.

[19] Mavrofrides EC, Cruz-Villegas V, Puliafito CA. (2004). Miscellaneous retinal diseases. In: Schuman JS, Puliafito CA, Fujimoto JG, eds. Optical coherence tomography of ocular diseases. Thorofare, NJ: SLACK, Inc.; 2004:457-482.

[20] Kang SW, Park CY, Ham DI. (2004). The correlation between fluorescein angiographic and optical coherence tomographic features in clinically significant diabetic macular edema. Am J Ophthalmol, Vol. 137, No. 2, (Feb), pp.313-322.

[21] Mavrofrides EC, Rogers AH, Truong S et al. (2005). Vitroretinal interface disorders. In: Schuman JS, Puliafito CA, Fujimoto JG, eds. Optical coherence tomography of ocular diseases. Thorofare, NJ: SLACK, Inc.; 2005: 57-102.

[22] Mori K, Gehlbach PL, Sano A, Deguchi T, Yoneya S. (2004). Comparison of epiretinal membranes of differing pathogenesis using optical coherence tomography. Retina, Vol. 24, No. 1, (Feb), pp. 57-62.

[23] Eriksson U, Larsson E, Holmstrom G. (2004). Optical coherence tomography in the diagnosis of juvenile X-linked retinoschisis. Acta Ophthalmol Scand, Vol. 82, No. 2, (Apr), pp. 218-23.

[24] Dawczynski J, Koenigsdoerffer E, Augsten R, Strobel J. (2007). Anterior optical coherence tomography: a non-contact technique for anterior chamber evaluation. Graefe's Arch Clin. Exp. Ophthalmol., Vol. 245, No. 3, pp. 423–425.

[25] Tan AN, Sauren LDC, de Brabander J et al. (2011). Reproducibility of anterior chamber angle measurements with anterior segment optical coherence tomography. Invest. Ophthalmol. Vis. Sci, Vol. 52, No. 5, pp. 2095–2099.

[26] Milla M, Piñero DP, Amparo F, Alió JL. (2011). Pachymetric measurements with a new Scheimpflug photography-based system: intraobserver repeatability and agreement with optical coherence tomography pachymetry. J. Cataract Refract. Surg, Vol. 37, No. 2, pp. 310–316.

[27] Nakagawa T, Maeda N, Higashiura R et al. (2011). Corneal topographic analysis in patients with keratoconus using 3-dimensional anterior segment optical coherence tomography. J. Cataract Refract. Surg, Vol. 37, No. 10, pp. 1871–1878.

[28] Baïkoff G, Lutun E, Wei J, Ferraz C. (2004). Anterior chamber optical coherence tomography study of human natural accommodation in a 19-year-old albino. J. Cataract Refract. Surg, Vol. 30, No. 3, pp. 696–701.

[29] Baïkoff G, Lutun E, Ferraz C, Wei J. (2004). Static and dynamic analysis of the anterior segment with optical coherence tomography. J. Cataract Refract. Surg, Vol. 30, No. 9, pp. 1843–1850.

[30] Dinc U, Gorgun E, Oncel B et al. (2010). Assessment of anterior chamber depth using visante optical coherence tomography, slitlamp optical coherence tomography, IOL master, pentacam and orbscan II. Ophthalmologica, Vol. 224, No. 6, pp. 341–346.

[31] Mamalis N. (2010). Phakic intraocular lenses. J. Cataract Refract. Surg, Vol. 36, No. 11, pp. 1805–1806.

[32] Lindland A, Heger H, Kugelberg M, Zetterström C. (2010). Vaulting of myopic and toric implantable collamer lenses during accommodation measured with Visante optical coherence tomography. Ophthalmology,Vol. 117, No. 6, pp. 1245–1250.

[33] Jagow von B, Kohnen T. (2009). Corneal architecture of femtosecond laser and microkeratome flaps imaged by anterior segment optical coherence tomography. J. Cataract Refract. Surg, Vol. 35, No. 1, pp. 35–41.

[34] Can I, Bayhan HA, Celik H, Bostancı CB. (2011). Anterior segment optical coherence tomography evaluation and comparison of main clear corneal incisions in microcoaxial and biaxial cataract surgery. J. Cataract Refract. Surg, Vol. 37, No. 3, pp. 490–500.

[35] Torres LF, Saez-Espinola F, Colina JM et al. (2006). In vivo architectural analysis of 3.2 mm clear corneal incisions for phacoemulsification using optical coherence tomography. J. Cataract Refract. Surg, Vol. 32, No. 37, pp. 1820–1826.

[36] Fukuda S, Kawana K, Yasuno Y, Oshika T. (2011). Wound architecture of clear corneal incision with or without stromal hydration observed with 3-dimensional optical coherence tomography. Am. J. Ophthalmol, Vol. 151, No. 3, pp. 413–419.

[37] Kymionis GD, Ide T, Donaldson K, Yoo SH. (2010). Diagnosis of donor graft partial dislocation behind the iris after DSAEK with anterior segment OCT. Ophthalmic

Surg. Lasers Imaging Vol. 9, pp. 1–2. Mar 9 :1-2 doi 10.3928/15428877.20100215-14[Epub ahead of print]

[38] Ide T, Yoo SH, Kymionis G, Shah P. (2008). Double Descemet's membranes after penetrating keratoplasty with anterior segment optical coherence tomography. Ophthalmic Surg. Lasers Imaging, Vol. 39, No. 5, pp. 422–425.

[39] Kymionis GD, Suh LH, Dubovy SR, Yoo SH. (2007). Diagnosis of residual Descemet's membrane after Descemet's stripping endothelial keratoplasty with anterior segment optical coherence tomography. J. Cataract Refract. Surg, Vol. 33, No. 7, pp. 1322–1324.

[40] Suh LH, Yoo SH, Deobhakta A et al. (2008). Complications of Descemet's stripping with automated endothelial keratoplasty: survey of 118 eyes at One Institute. Ophthalmology, Vol. 115, No. 9, pp. 1517–1524.

[41] Yoo SH, Kymionis GD, Deobhakta AA et al. (2008). One-year results and anterior segment optical coherence tomography findings of Descemet stripping automated endothelial keratoplasty combined with phacoemulsification. Arch Ophthalmol, Vol. 126, No. 8, pp. 1052–1055.

[42] Stahl JE, Durrie DS, Schwendeman FJ, Boghossian AJ. (2007). Anterior segment OCT analysis of thin IntraLase femtosecond flaps. J. Refract. Surg, Vol. 23, No. 6, pp. 555–558.

[43] Hoffart L, Proust H, Matonti F, Conrath J, Ridings B. (2009). Correction of postkeratoplasty astigmatism by femtosecond laser compared with mechanized astigmatic keratotomy. Am. J. Ophthalmol, Vol. 147, No. 5, pp. 779–787.

[44] Nubile M, Carpineto P, Lanzini M et al. (2009). Femtosecond laser arcuate keratotomy for the correction of high astigmatism after keratoplasty. Ophthalmology, Vol. 116, No. 6, pp. 1083–1092.

[45] Yoo SH, Hurmeric V. (2011). Femtosecond laser-assisted keratoplasty. Am J Ophthalmol, Vol. 151, No. 2, pp. 190–191.

[46] Yoo S, Kymionis GD, Koreishi A et al. (2008). Femtosecond laser-assisted sutureless anterior lamellar keratoplasty. Ophthalmology Vol. 115, No. 8, pp. 1303–1307.

[47] Li Y, Netto M, Shekhar R, Krueger R, Huang D. (2007). A longitudinal study of LASIK flap and stromal thickness with high-speed optical coherence tomography. Ophthalmology Vol. 114, No. 6, pp. 1124–1132.

[48] Rosas SCH, Li Y, Zhang X et al. (2011). Repeatability of laser in situ keratomileusis flap thickness measurement by Fourier-domain optical coherence tomography. J. Cataract Refract. Surg, Vol. 37, No. 4, pp. 649–654.

[49] Kymionis GD, Ide T, Galor A, Yoo SH. (2009). Femtosecond-assisted anterior lamellar corneal staining-tattooing in a blind eye with leukocoria. Cornea, Vol. 28, No. 2, pp. 211–213.

[50] Kanellopoulos AJ. (2009). Collagen cross-linking in early keratoconus with riboflavin in a femtosecond laser-created pocket: initial clinical results. J. Refract. Surg, Vol. 25, No. 11, pp. 1034–1037.

[51] Nagy Z, Takacs A, Filkorn T, Sarayba M. (2009). Initial clinical evaluation of an intraocular femtosecond laser in cataract surgery. J. Refract. Surg, Vol. 25, No. 12, pp. 1053–1060.

[52] William WC, Juan FB, Rafael F et al. (2011). Facilitation of nuclear cataract removal by femtosecond laser pretreatment. ASCRS, (Abstract 982342).

[53] Wang J, Jiao S, Ruggeri M, Shousha MA, Chen Q. (2009). In situ visualization of tears on contact lens using ultra high resolution optical coherence tomography. Eye Contact Lens, Vol. 35, No. 2, pp. 44–49.

[54] Dayani PN, Maldonado R, Farsiu S, Toth CA. (2009). Intraoperative use of handheld spectral domain optical coherence tomography imaging in macular surgery. Retina, Vol. 29, No. 10, pp. 1457–1468.

[55] Christopoulos V, Kagemann L, Wollstein G, et al. (2007). In vivo corneal high–speed, ultra high resolution optical coherence tomography. Arch Ophthalmol, Vol. 125, No . 8, pp. 1027-35.

[56] Jeremy ZK, Carol LK, Shousha MA, Galor A, Rodrigo AH, Dubovy SR et al. (2012). Ultra–High Resolution optical coherence tomography for differentiation of ocular surface squamous neoplasia and pterygia. Ophthalmology, Vol. 119: No. 3, (Mar), pp. 481-486.

[57] Jiang C, Li Yan, Huang D, Brian AF. (2012). Study of Anterior Chamber Aqueous tube shunt by Fourier–Domain Optical coherence tomography. Journal of Ophthalmology, doi:10.1155/2012/189580

[58] Nordan LT, Slade SG, Baker RN, Suarez C, Juhasz T, Kurtz R. (2003). Femtosecond laser flap creation for laser in situ keratomileusis: six-month follow-up of initial U.S. clinical series. J. Refract. Surg, Vol. 19, No. 1, pp. 8–14.

[59] Seider M, Ide T, Kymionis GD, Culbertson WW, O'Brien T, Yoo S. (2008). Epithelial breakthrough during IntraLase flap creation for laser in situ keratomileusis. J. Cataract Refract. Surg, Vol. 34, No. 5, pp. 859–863.

[60] Ide T, Yoo SH, Kymionis GD, Haft P, O'Brien TP. (2009). Second femtosecond laser pass for incomplete laser in situ keratomileusis flaps caused by suction loss. J. Cataract Refract. Surg, Vol. 35, No. 1, pp. 153–157.

[61] Ide T, Wang J, Tao A et al. (2010). Intraoperative use of three-dimensional spectral-domain optical coherence tomography. Ophthalmic Surg. Lasers Imaging, Vol. 41, No. 2, pp. 250–254.

[62] Villate N, Mavrofrides EC, Davis J. (2004). Chorioretinal inflammatory diseases. In: Schuman JS, Puliafito CA, Fujimoto JG, eds. Optical coherence tomography of ocular diseases. Thorofare, NJ: SLACK, Inc.; 2004:371-412.

[63] Suzuki T, Terasaki H, Niwa T. (2003). Optical coherence tomography and focal macular electroretinogram in eyes with epiretinal membrane and macular pseudohole. Am J Ophthalmol, Vol. 136, No. 1, (Jul), pp. 62-67

[64] Massin P, Allouch C, Haouchine B, Metge F, Pâques M, et al. (2000). Optical coherence tomography of idiopathic macular epiretinal membranes before and after surgery. Am J Ophthalmol, Vol. 130, No. 6, (Dec), pp. 732-739.

[65] Antcliff RJ, Stanford MR, Chauhan DS, Graham EM, Spalton DJ, et al. (2002). Comparison between Optical coherence tomography and fundus fluorescein angiography for the detection of cystoid macular edema in patients with uveitis. Ophthalmology, Vol. 107, No. 3, (Mar), pp. 593-599.

[66] Markomichelakis NN, Halkiadakis I, Pantelia E, Peponis V, Patelis A, et al. (2004). Patterns of macular edema in patients with uveitis: qualitative and quantitative assessment using Optical coherence tomography. Ophthalmology, Vol. 111, No. 5, (May), pp. 946-953.

[67] Schaudig UH, Glaefke C, Scholz F, Richard G. (2000). Optical coherence tomography for retinal thickness measurement in diabetic patients without clinically significant macular edema. Ophthalm Surg Lasers, Vol. 31, No. 3, (May-Jun) pp. 182-186.

[68] Marmor MF. (2012). Comparison of screening procedures in hydroxychloroquine toxicity. Arch Ophthalmol, Vol. 130, No. 4, pp. 461-9

[69] Korah S, Kuriakose T. (2008). Optical coherence tomography in a patient with chloroquine-induced maculopathy. Indian J Ophthalmol, Vol. 56, No. 6, (Nov-Dec), pp. 511-3

[70] Hager T, Hoffmann S, Seitz B. (2010). Unusual symptoms for tamoxifen –associated maculopathy. Ophthalmologe, Vol. 107, No. 8, pp. 750-2.

[71] Menon V, Jain D, Saxena R, Sood R. (2009). Prospective evaluation of visual function for early detection of ethambutol toxicity. Br J Ophthalmol, Vol. 93, No. 9, pp. 1251-4

[72] Moseng L, Saeter M, Mørch-Johnsen GH, Hoff JM, Gajda A, Brodtkorb E, et al. (2011). Retinal nerve fibre layer attenuation: clinical indicator for vigabatrin toxicity. Acta Ophthalmol, Vol. 89, No. 5, pp. 452-8.

[73] Coscas F, Coscas G, Zucchiatti I, Bandello F, Soubrane G, Souied E. (2012). Optical coherence tomography in tadalafil-associated retinal toxicity. Eur J Ophthalmol, Feb7:0.doi:10.5301/ejo.5000127.

[74] Rogers AH, Martidis A, Greenberg PB, Puliafito CA. (2002). Optical coherence tomography findings following photodynamic therapy of choroidal neovascularisation. Am J Ophthalmol, Vol. 134, No. 4, (Oct), pp. 566-576.

[75] Decroos FC, Toth CA, Folgar FA, Pakola S, Stinnett SS, Heydary CS, et al. (2012). Characterization of vitreoretinal interface disorders using OCT in the interventional phase 3 trials of ocriplasmin. Invest Ophthalmol Vis Sci. (Aug 9). [Epub ahead of print]

[76] Stalmans P, Delaey C, de Smet MD, van Dijkman E, Pakola S. (2010). Intravitreal injection of microplasmin for treatment of vitreomacular adhesion: results of a prospective, randomized, sham-controlled phase II trial (the MIVI-IIT trial). Retina, Vol. 30, No. 7, pp. 1122-7.

[77] Jumper JM, Gallemore RP, McCuen BW 2nd, Toth CA. (2000). Features of macular hole closure in the early postoperative period using optical coherence tomography. Retina, Vol. 20, No. 3, pp. 232-237.

[78] Sato H, Kawasaki R, Yamashita H. (2003). Observation of idiopathic full-thickness macular hole closure in early postoperative period as evaluated by optical coherence tomography. Am J Ophthalmol, Vol. 136, No. 1, (Jul), pp. 185-187.

[79] Chavala SH, Farsiu S, Maldonado R ,Wallace DK, Freedman SF ,Toth CA. (2009). Insights into advanced retinopathy of prematurity using handheld spectral domain optical coherence tomography. Ophthalmology Vol. 116, No. 12, pp. 2448 -2456

[80] Vinekar A, Sivakumar M, Shetty R, et al. (2010). A novel technique using spectral domain optical coherence tomography (Spectralis, SD-OCT+HRA) to image supine non –anaesthetized infants: utility demonstrated in aggressive posterior retinopathy of prematurity. Eye, Vol. 24, No. 2, pp. 379-382

[81] Muni RH, Kohly RP, Charonis AC, Lee TC. (2010). Retinoschisis detected with handheld spectral domain optical coherence tomography in neonates with advanced retinopathy of prematurity. Arch Ophthalmol, Vol. 128, No. 1, pp. 57-62

[82] Maldonado RS, Izatt JA, Sarin N, et al. (2010). Optimizing handheld spectral domain optical coherence tomography imaging for neonates and infants and children. Invest. Ophthalmol. Vis. Sci. Vol. 51, No. 5, pp. 2678 -2685.

[83] Lee AC, Maldonado RS , Sarin N, et al. (2011). Macular features from spectral domain optical coherence tomography as an adjunct to indirect ophthalmoscopy in retinopathy of prematurity. Retina, Vol. 31, No.8, pp. 1470 -1482

[84] Maldonado RS, O' Connell RV, Sarin N, et al. (2011). Dynamics of human foveal development after premature birth. Ophthalmology, Vol. 118, No.12, (Dec), pp. 2315-25.

[85] Vinekar A, Avadhani K, Sivakumar M et al. (2011). Understanding clinically undetected macular changes in early retinopathy of prematurity on spectral domain optical coherence tomography. Invest. Ophthalmol. Vis. Sci. Vol. 52, No.8, (Aug), pp. 5183-5188

[86] Maldonado RS, O' Connell R, Ascher SB, Sarin N, Freedman SF, et al. (2012). Spectral –domain optical coherence tomographic assessment of severity of cystoid macular

edema in retinopathy of prematurity. Arch Ophthalmol, Vol.130, No. 5, (May), pp. 569 -78

[87] Wang XM, Cui DM, Yang X, Huo LJ, Liu X, et al.(2012). Characteristics of the macula in amblyopic eyes by optical coherence tomography. Int J Ophthalmol, Vol. 5, No. 2, pp.172-176.

Chapter 2

B-Scan and 'En-Face'Spectral-Domain Optical Coherence Tomography Imaging for the Diagnosis and Follow-Up of White Dot Syndromes

Benjamin Wolff, Alexandre Matet, Vivien Vasseur,
José-Alain Sahel and Martine Mauget-Faÿsse

Additional information is available at the end of the chapter

http://dx.doi.org/10.5772/53959

1. Introduction

The term 'white dot syndromes' (WDS) refers to several inflammatory diseases of the retina and choroid caused by immune dysregulation. They consist of the following disorders, with overlapping clinical features:

- Acute posterior multifocal placoid pigment epitheliopathy (APMPPE)
- Serpiginous choroidopathy
- Multiple evanescent white dot syndrome (MEWDS)
- Birdshot retinochoroidopathy
- Acute retinal pigment epitheliitis (ARPE)
- Multifocal choroiditis and panuveitis syndrome (MCP)
- Punctuate inner choroidopathy (PIC), and
- Acute zonal occult outer retinopathy (AZOOR)

These conditions usually occur following an influenza-like illness, but their patho-physiologic mechanism remains poorly understood. The white dot syndromes affect more frequently young females and individuals with mild myopia, and present as white or yellow, deep, round lesions in the central fundus. Their size and number can vary between each entity, as well as their uni- or bilateral involvement.

In addition to these clinical parameters, fluorescein (FA) and indocyanine green angiographies (ICGA) help in identifying the diagnosis [1]. They also help assess the level of inflammatory activity and detect complications.

The high resolution of the scans generated by Spectral Domain Optical Coherence Tomography (SD-OCT) offers a helpful tool in the management of WDS. SD-OCT allows a direct, non-contact visualization of involved retinal layers and thereby provides information concerning the:

- accurate location of the inflammatory process
- integrity of the photoreceptors inner segment / outer segment junction (IS/OS)
- course of the inflammatory process, leading to resolution or residual scarring
- presence of complications such as neovascularization

Moreover, the use of 'en-face' OCT for WDS allows a layer-by-layer view of the involved retina. This novel imaging technique generates frontal scans derived from SD-OCT.

The scans of "en face" OCT imaging of WDS were obtained by Spectral-domain OCT (Spectralis® Heidelberg Engineering, Heidelberg, Germany). For every case, the macula was analyzed using SD-OCT (Spectralis® Heidelberg Engineering, Heidelberg, Germany) and macular mapping consisting of 197 transverse sections in a 5.79 x 5.79 mm^2 central retinal area. Tridimensional reconstruction generated by the pooling of these sections provides a virtual macular brick, through which 496 shifting sections in the coronal plane result in the C-scan, or "en face" OCT.

In contrast, B-scans for conventional OCT are derived from sagittal and transverse sections. Enhanced depth imaging OCT (EDI-OCT) is a new tool that improves the sensitivity of the imaging in deeper layers of retinal tissue. The visualization of the choroid is increased and thus the obtained measurements are more accurate.

For each condition belonging to the WDS, we compared the results from SD-OCT "B-scan" and 'en-face' with data from classical retinal imaging, namely fundus photography and angiography.

2. MEWDS, Multiple evanescent white dot syndrome (figure 1)

MEWDS typically affects young females, and presents as a sudden visual loss with paracentral scotomas. In 80% of cases the condition remains unilateral. Fundus examination reveals small, discrete perifoveolar dots, very mild vitritis, and, in some cases, papillitis. On fluorescein angiography these dots appear hyperfluorescent, but are hypofluorescent on ICGA. The natural history leads usually to complete and spontaneous resolution within weeks.

- SD-OCT at the acute stage identifies the lesions in the outer retina as hyperreflective thickened lesions of the inner segment/outer segment (IS/OS) junction, alternating with disruption of the IS/OS junction [2]. Small highly reflective dots involving the RPE inner layer, the IS/OS junction and the outer nuclear layer can be observed. EDI-OCT frequently demonstrates choroidal thickening.

- 'En-face' OCT shows multifocal involvement in the plane of the IS-OS junction, consisting of various round hyporeflective lesions alternating with large hyperreflective areas. Centrally, they may appear as confluent, which explains the "moth-eaten" appearance of the macula in some cases. Hypofluorescent spots on ICGA and IS-OS disruption zones on 'en-face' OCT are well correlated [3]. This correlation is also observed between SD-OCT B-scans and ICGA.

During follow-up, a progressive and complete restitution of outer retinal layers is observed. This observation is correlated with functional resolution [4]. However, focal gaps in IS/OS junction may persist in some cases and are associated with central visual field defects.

3. Acute posterior multifocal placoid pigment epitheliopathy (APMPPE) (figure 2 and 3)

In this bilateral, often asymmetrical condition, that presents in healthy young adults, with both male and female being affected equally, fundus examination reveals yellowish-white plaques of 1 to 2 disc diameters, scattered from the fovea to the equator [5]. They may be associated with mild vitritis. Their FA appearance in the acute stage is pathognomonic: early blockade hypofluorescence, followed by late hyperfluorescence caused by staining. ICGA shows multiple lesions that may be confluent, and that remain hypofluorescent during all angiographic stages.

In the acute stage, SD-OCT shows:

- On B-scan: hyperreflective lesions in outer retinal layers, some extending to Henle's fibers layer. Irregularities in IS/OS, external limiting membrane, and inner pigment epithelium layer are also visible around those highly reflective lesions [6]. In the acute phase, an elevation of the IS/OS junction with subretinal fluid located between this layer and the RPE may be observed. In severe cases, this hyporeflective space between the IS/OS and external limiting membrane can mimic an encapsulated serous retinal detachment. Hyperreflective intrachoroidal spots are seen on EDI mode, suggesting choroidal inflammation.
- On 'en-face' OCT: the extent of the selesions, located in the external nuclear layer, are well defined. These lesions perfectly match the hypofluorescent plaques seen on ICGA. In severe cases with encapsulated serous retinal detachment, 'en-face' OCT reveals a wide hyporeflective lesion with hyperreflective borders. These large hyporeflective lesions may contain tiny reflective deposits.

In the late stages, SD-OCT shows:

- On B-scans: retinal thinning with disruption of the IS/OS and inner pigment epithelium, located where hyperreflective lesions had been observed. Irregular or focal gaps in external

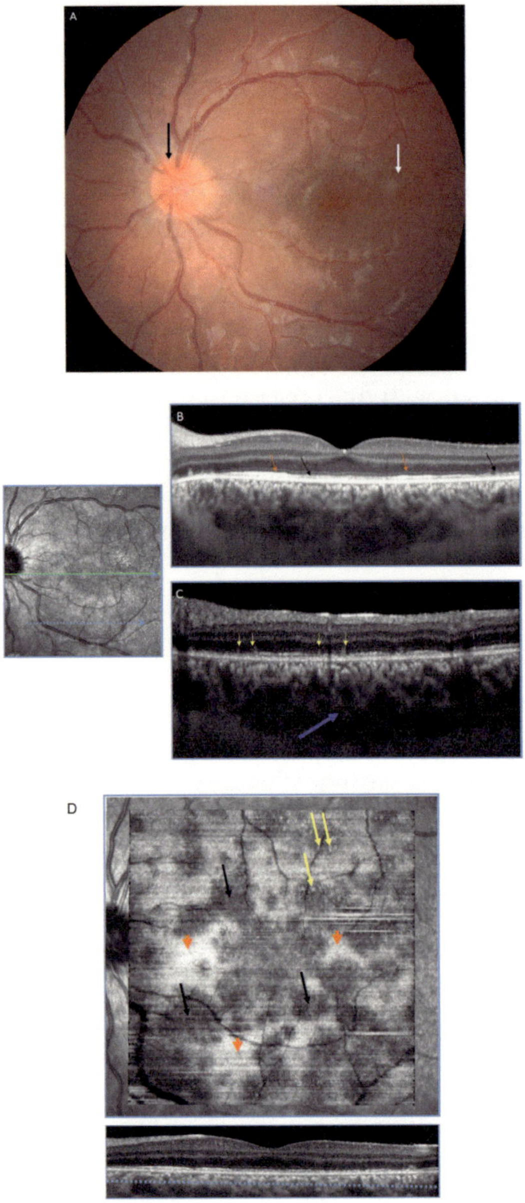

Figure 1. MEWDS.a) MEWD acute phase: color fundus photography. Unilateral (Left eye) discrete perifoveal dots (white arrow) with light papillitis(black arrow), b) MEWDS acute phase: SD-OCT B-scan. Visualization of large IS/OS segment disruptions (black arrow) in the posterior pole, mostly in the foveal region, alternating with few focal, highly hyperreflective, thickened IS/OS zones (orange arrows). c) MEWDS acute phase: SD-OCT B-scan. Tiny hyperreflective elevations (spicules) (yellow arrows) visible in the areas with IS/OS disruption. Note the significant choroidal thickening (blue arrow).d) MEWDS acute phase: En Face OCT. Multifocal involvement in the plane of the IS-OS junction, consisting of various round or oval coalescing hyporeflective lesions (black arrows) corresponding to areas of disrupted IS/OS junctions seen on B-scans, alternating with large hyperreflective areas (orange arrows). The « spicules » are imaged as very small hyperreflective spots (yellow arrows) within the hyporeflective zones of IS/OS junction disruptions.

http://dx.doi.org/10.5772/53959

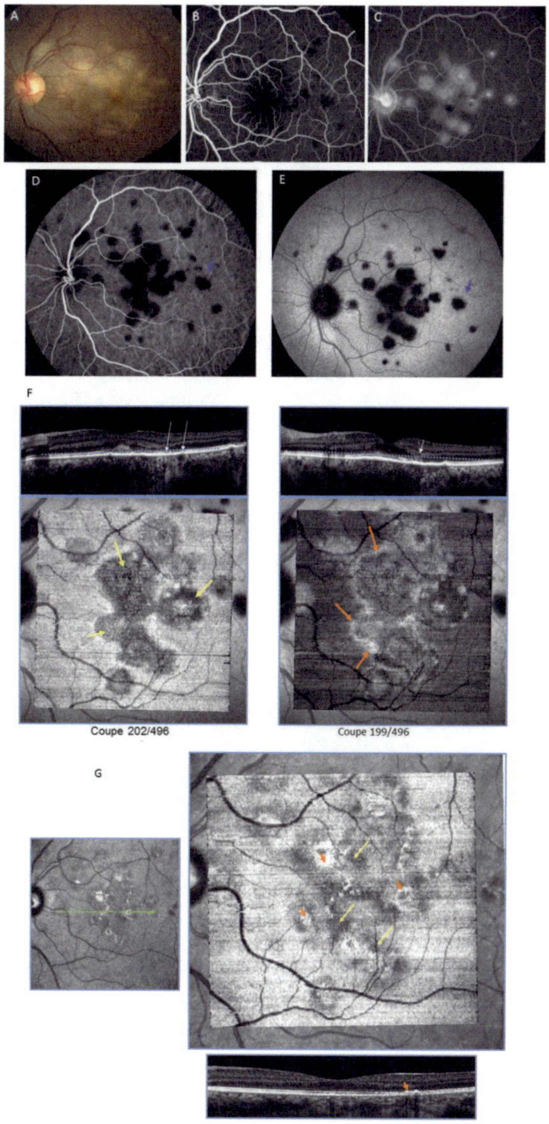

Figure 2. AMPPE.(a-e). AMPPE early phase: a: AMPPE typical presentation with yellowish-white plaques of 1 to 2 disc diameters, scattered from the fovea to the equator on color fundus photography. FA appearance in the acute phase is pathognomonic with early blockade hypofluorescence, (figure 2b)followed by late hyperfluorescence phase (figure 2c). ICGA shows multiple lesions that may be confluent, and that remain hypofluorescent during all angiographic phases (early phase: figure 2d) and late phase (figure 2e). f) AMPPE early phase: SD-OCT B-scan both images. Top: Hyperreflective lesions in the outer retinal layers, some extending to Henle's fibers layer. Irregularities in the IS/OS, external limiting membrane, and inner pigment epithelium layer are seen around the hyperreflective lesions (white arrows). Bottom: En face OCT. Left: Visualization of the hyporeflective lesions corresponding to the alterations in the IS/OS junction (yellow arrows). Right: Hyperreflective band within the outer nuclear layer (orange arrows) surrounding the hyporeflective lesions (corresponding to hypofluorescent spots on ICGA).g) AMPPE late phase.Left: SD-OCT B-scan. Areas of irregularly thickened pigment epithelium (orange arrow). Right: En face OCT. These irregularly thickened areas of pigment epithelium are visualized as hyperreflective zones (orange arrows).Hyporeflective areas are due to previous IS/OS junction involvement (yellow arrows).

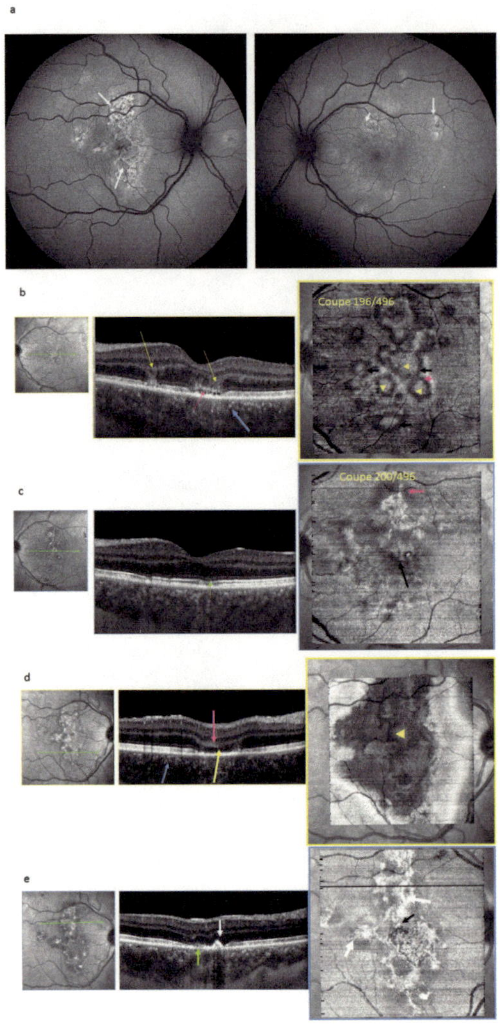

Figure 3. AMPPE.a) AMPPE early phase of a more severe case. Autofluorescence images: Irregular autofluorescent areas in both eyes (white arrows). b) AMPPE early phase, left eye. Left: SD-OCT B-scan. Hyperreflective lesions (yellow arrows) in the outer retinal layers, extending to Henle's fibers layer. Irregularities in the IS/OS, external limiting membrane, and inner pigment epithelium layers are visible around the highly reflective lesions. Subretinal fluid is observed located between the IS/OS junction and the RPE (pink arrow) as well as hyperreflective small spots within the choroid (blue arrows). Right: En face OCT. Round or oval coalescing moderately reflective lesions (yellow arrow head) bordered by a hyporeflective band (black arrows) located inside a hyperreflective area (pink arrow head). c) AMPPE late phase. Left: SD-OCT B-scan. Thinned IS/OS junction areas and RPE irregularities (green arrows) Right: En face OCT. Global improvement at the IS/OS junction plane with scarring represented by hyper- (pink arrows) and hyporeflective areas (black arrows) d) AMPPE early phase. Left: SD-OCT B-scan. Severe alterations of the whole outer retina (pink arrows) with IS/OS segment disruption (yellow arrow) and hyperreflective spots within the choroid (blue arrow). Right: En face OCT. Scan at the level of IS/OS segment plane: extensive hyporeflective lesions (yellow arrow head) corresponding to IS/OS segment disruption. e). AMPPE late phase. Left: SD-OCT B-scan. Outer retinal scar represented by alternation of thinning (green arrow) and thickening (white arrow) of the IS/OS and RPE tissues. Right: En face OCT. Global improvement at the IS/OS plane with the association of hyperreflective (white arrows) and hyporeflective areas (black arrow) of the scarring process in the IS/OS and RPE complex.

limiting membrane can also occur [7]. In some cases, complete resolution of outer retinal defects may be seen. Classically, involvement of the pigment epithelium has been described [8]. It appears in the late stage as areas of irregular, thickened pigment epithelium.

- 'En-face' OCT demonstrates a decrease in the highly reflective lesions that are replaced with hyporeflective areas due to IS/OS junction involvement. Hyperreflective dots corresponding to focal areas of thickened RPE can be observed inside this hyporeflective IS/OS junction layer.

4. Serpiginous choroiditis (figure 4)

This chronic, progressive, bilateral and asymmetrical condition presents equally in men and women, from the 2nd to the 6th decade of life [9]. Various infectious etiologies have been suggested, among which tuberculosis must be formally ruled out [10]. Clinical and angiographic examination identifies greyish-white digitations starting from the optic disc. Its active border appears hypofluorescent on FA. ICGA is a useful tool for evaluating the response to treatment, since lesions are more extended on ICGA than on FA.

- On SD-OCT, in the active phase, hyperreflective lesions in the outer retinal layers can be observed, some extending to Henle's fibers layer. In the late stage, areas of irregular, thickened pigment epithelium are seen regarding a loss of structure in the external layers (IS/OS, Verhoeff's membrane) [11]. Many hyperreflective dots are present inside the choroid. Choroidal thickening is also seen on EDI.

- 'En-face' OCT confirms that the appearance of the network of digitations is due to outer retinal changes [12]. Active lesions are observed at the level of the ONL as branching mildly reflective lesions. In the late stage, hyperreflective digitations are seen at the level of the RPE and correspond to areas of thickened RPE.

5. Punctuate inner choroiditis (PIC) and multifocal choroiditis and panuveitis (MCP) (figure 5)

These two conditions share common characteristics: small, sharp lesions that evolve rapidly towards pigmented scars, affecting myopic females between 20 and 40 years of age. PIC differs from MCP by the absence of vitritis and the limitation of the lesions to the posterior fundus, while they can extend to the equatorial fundus in MCP [13]. FA is marked by a late hyperfluorescence. From mid-sequence on ICGA, the lesions appear hypofluorescent, and more numerous than on funduscopy.

- With SD-OCT, sections through a lesion show accumulation of drusenoid deposits between the pigment epithelium and Bruch's membrane [14]. Disruption of the IS/OS junction and RPE may be observed on the top of these elevations.

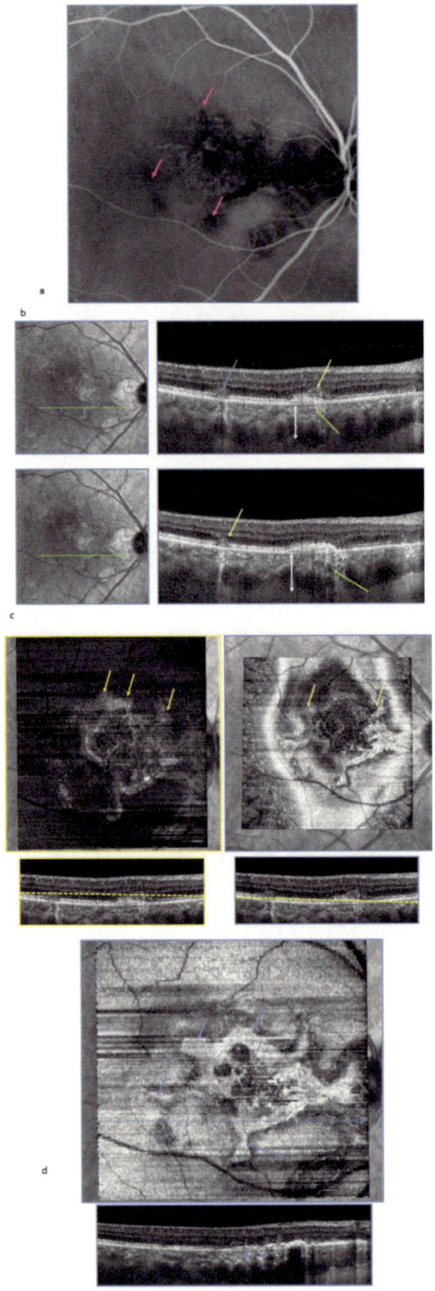

Figure 4. SERPIGINOUS CHOROIDITIS. a) Serpiginous choroiditis acute phase: ICGA. Hypo fluorescent digitations starting from the optic disc (pink arrows). b) Serpiginous choroiditis acute phase: SD-OCT (top and down) Hyperreflective lesions in the outer retinal layers, some extending to Henle's fibers layer (yellow arrows). Numerous hyperreflective dots are present inside the choroid (green arrows). Choroidal thickening is seen on EDI (white double head arrow). c) Serpiginous choroiditis acute phase: Active lesions are observed at the level of the ONL (left) and IS/OS junction layer (right) as branching mildly reflective lesions (yellow arrows). d) Serpiginous choroiditis late phase: in the late stage, hyperreflective digitations are seen at the level of the RPE and correspond to areas of thickened RPE (blue arrows).

http://dx.doi.org/10.5772/53959

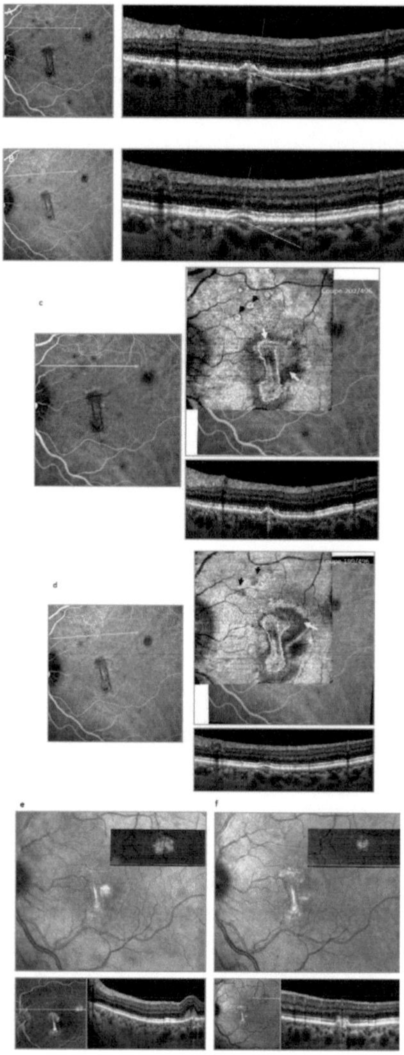

Figure 5. CMF.a) CMF acute phase: SD-OCT B-scan. Presence of deposits between the Brüch's membrane and RPE looking like fusiform, hyperreflective, small, dome shape elevations of the RPE (green arrows). An interruption of the IS/OS junction at the top of the dome shape elevation is also seen (pink arrow) b) CMF late phase: SD-OCT B-scan, Post treatment: the RPE elevation slowly and progressively decreases after treatment (green arrow) with the disappearance of the interruptions in the IS/OS junction (pink arrow). c) CMF acute phase: En Face OCT. Multiple, small, round or oval shaped hyperreflective lesions are seen in front of the RPE layer with a well defined hyporeflective centre and borders (black arrows).In the fovea, the hyperreflective CNV scar (with a hyperreflective border) is fibrous but still active (white arrow) with a hyporeflective area all around the scar corresponding to a serous retinal detachment(yellow arrow). d) CMF late phase: En Face OCT. Progressive disappearance of the outer retinal lesions which are faintly hyporeflective (black arrows). However, the CNV is still active (yellow arrow) e). Differentiation between CNV and choroiditis lesion. En face OCT, before anti-VEGF treatment: the moderately hyperreflective CNV has irregular edges. It corresponds on SD-OCT B-scan to the moderately hyperreflective pre- epithelial lesion associated with overlying retinal thickening. f). Differentiation between CNV and choroiditis lesion. En face OCT, after anti-VEGF treatment: the borders of the CNV become more hyperreflective and better defined.This corresponds on SD-OCT B-scan to an involuted CNV that has become more hyperreflective but still active (blurred limits in the superior part).

- In the macular area, 'en-face' OCT shows the presence of multiple hyperreflective lesions above the level of the pigment epithelium. These lesions often show mild central hyporeflectivity. Comparison of 'en-face' OCT with ICGA reveals that these highly reflective lesions and hypofluorescent dots on ICGA closely match. This correlation is also observed with SD-OCT B-scans.

During follow-up, these outer retinal lesions progressively regress on 'en-face' OCT, which is usually associated with functional recovery.

Both PIC and MCP are at high risk of neovascular complications.

- When neovascularization occurs, a fusiform, hyperreflective thickening above the level of the pigment epithelium is seen on SD-OCT B-scans, and is usually associated with intraretinal cystoid exudative cavities [15].
- 'En-face' OCT imaging of this lesion, above the level of the pigment epithelium, reveals its irregular borders, thus distinguishing it from inflammatory lesions. 'En-face' OCT also allows analysis of all exudative cavities in one section, which is helpful for an improved, comparative follow-up.

This neovascularization can regress after repeated intravitreal anti-VEGF injections, providing that inflammation is sufficiently controlled.

6. Birdshot chorioretinopathy (figure 6)

Birdshot chorioretinopathy is a slowly progressing, bilateral inflammation. It predominantly affects women and appears between 30 and 70 (mean age: 53) years. Association with HLA A29 is a common feature. Multiple hypopigmented choroidal lesions characterize the fundus [17]. FA is more useful in detecting complications (vasculitis, macular edema) than in analyzing the dots, for which ICGA is preferred. Indeed, they appear hypopigmented and often more numerous than on funduscopy.

- During active and severe phases, SD-OCT may identify drusenoid deposits between the pigment epithelium and IS/OS junction with a posterior shadow inside the choroid. Hyperreflective intraretinal dots, located in the outer nuclear layer (ONL) and corresponding to inflammatory deposits may be seen in acute phase. However, SD-OCT's main application for Birdshot chorioretinopathy is the screening for complications, mostly cystoid macular edema [18] or epiretinal membrane [19]. In the late phase, cases with poor control of inflammation (due to insufficient treatment or lack of response to appropriate therapy) evolve towards outer retinal atrophy, with IS/OS disruptions. SD-OCT is then an efficient tool to distinguish between these various causes of visual loss, and leads to appropriate treatment when needed [20].
- On 'en face' OCT, a hyperreflective border stretching along the retinal vessels and corresponding to vasculitis can be observed. Multiple hyperreflective dots can be seen inside the ONL. In acute and severe phases, mildly reflective lesions located above the RPE layer can be seen. The selesions match hypofluorescent lesions observed with ICGA.

http://dx.doi.org/10.5772/53959

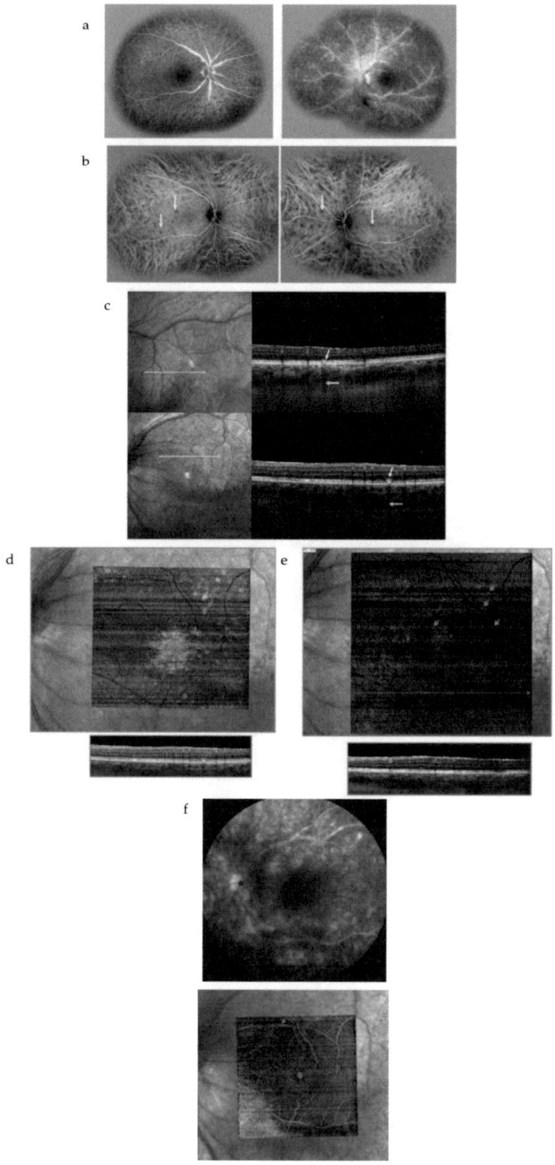

Figure 6. Birdshot chorioretinopathy. a) Birdshot chorioretinopathy, active phase: marked retinal vasculitis observed on FA with dye leakage at the level of the vascular wall (blue arrows). b) Birdshot chorioretinopathy, active phase. IC-GA: numerous hypofluorescent spots are visible scattered in the posterior pole and nasal to the optic nerve during all the angiography sequences (Yellow arrow). c) Birdshot chorioretinopathy, active phase. SD-OCT B-scan: small hyperreflective lesions (white arrows) are seen located inside the RPE behind the IS/OS and leading to a shadow cone (green arrow) at the choroidal level (drusenoid like deposits). d) En face OCT: Birdshot chorioretinopathy, severe clinical forms. Multiple hypermoderately hyperreflective spots are observed between the RPE and the IS/OS junction (blue arrows). e) Birdshot chorioretinopathy, active phase. En face OCT: small multiple hyperreflective spots are visualized in the outer nuclear layer (blue arrows). Corresponding b-scan in the bottom. f) Birdshot chorioretinopathy, active phase. Top: FA of a patient with moderate vasculitis. Bottom: « en face » OCT improves the visualization of vasculitis by the hyperreflective sheathing of the vascular wall (pink arrow).

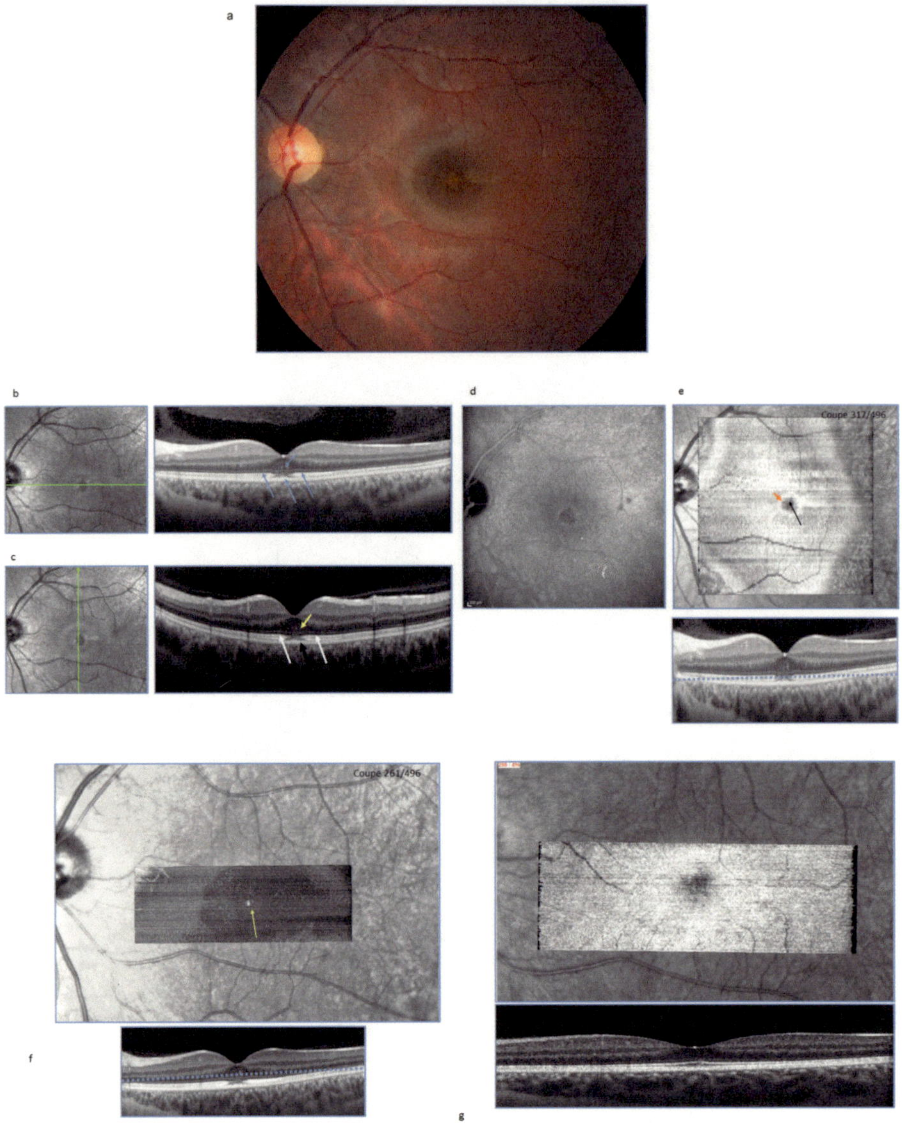

Figure 7. ARPE. a) ARPE acute phase: Yellowish halo around the fovea on color fundus photography. b and c. ARPE acute phase, horizontal and vertical SD-OCT B-scan crossing the fovea: disruption of both the internal RPE layer and IS/OS junction in the fovea (black arrows). Small hyperreflective foveal deposits (yellow arrow) are seen at the level of the internal nuclear layer. A faint hyperreflective IS/OS segment thickening is visualized around the central disruption (white arrows). d) ARPE early phase. Late phase ICGA shows mild hyperreflective halo (cockade shape) in the fovea. e). ARPE early phase, En face OCT: scan at the IS/OS junction plane. Hyperreflective halo (cockade shape) is visualized surrounding the fovea that appears hyporeflective (orange arrow). The halo corresponds to the faint hyperreflective thickening of the IS/OS junction around the hyporeflective central zone corresponding to the central IS/OS junction disruption (black arrow). f) ARPE early phase, En face OCT. Punctuate hyperreflective foveolar spots corresponding to the central deposits found in the acute phase at the outer nuclear layer level (yellow arrow).g) ARPE late phase, SD-OCT B-scan (top) and En face OCT (down): return to normality with incomplete recovery of the central IS/OS junction disruption.

7. Acute retinal pigment epitheliitis (ARPE) (figure 7)

ARPE, or Krill's disease, named after its first description by Krill in 1974 [21], is a benign, self-limited, bilateral yet asymmetrical condition affecting adults between 10 and 40 years of age. Funduscopy identifies a yellowish halo around the fovea, without vitritis. ICGA is crucial to rule out a MEWDS that may have a similar presentation. It shows a typical, sharply demarcated, round, macular area [22].

- A subfoveal involvement with blurring of the inner pigment epithelium and IS/OS junction is visible on SD-OCT. Small hyperreflective deposits between the IS/OS junction and outer nuclear layer are identified in some cases. Around this disrupted foveal area, one can frequently observe IS/OS junction thickening.
- The extent of outer retinal damage, mainly at IS/OS level, is evidenced by 'en-face' OCT. The central lesion demonstrates a cockade-like appearance with a hyporeflective center and a hyperreflective border. This cockade appearance matches the pattern observed on ICGA. Punctuate, highly reflective, subfoveolar lesions, resolving within days, can also be observed. During follow-up, full resolution of all the abnormal findings occurs without treatment [22].

8. Conclusion

White dots syndromes refer to several disease that evolve quickly. Retinal and choroidal involvement follows different phases: invasive phase, intermediate phase and chronic phase. Retinal and choroidal changes observed with multimodal imaging are transient and may disappear quickly in some cases. All these entities probably share a common pathway leading to external retinal involvement. 'En face' OCT imaging enables the assessment of the extent of structural damage occurring in WDS. OCT with "en face" OCT enhances its sensitivity, allowing earlier diagnosis of retinal changes and a more reliable follow-up. Further prospective studies including more patients will be necessary to confirm these results.

Author details

Benjamin Wolff*, Alexandre Matet, Vivien Vasseur, José-Alain Sahel and Martine Mauget-Faÿsse

*Address all correspondence to: bwolff@hotmail.fr

Professor Sahel Department, Rothschild Ophthalmologic Foundation, Paris, France

References

[1] Cohen SY, Dubois L, Quentel G, *et al.* Is indocyanine green angiography still relevant? Retina 2011;31:209–21.

[2] Nguyen MHT, Witkin AJ, Reichel E, *et al.* Microstructural abnormalities in MEWDS demonstrated by ultrahigh resolution optical coherence tomography. Retina 2007;27:414–8.

[3] Hangai M, Fujimoto M, Yoshimura N. Features and function of multiple evanescent white dot syndrome. Arch Ophthalmol 2009;127:1307–13.

[4] Li D, Kishi S. Restored photoreceptor outer segment damage in multiple evanescent white dot syndrome. Ophthalmology 2009;116:762–70.

[5] Fiore T, Iaccheri B, Androudi S, *et al.* Acute posterior multifocal placoid pigment epitheliopathy: outcome and visual prognosis. Retina 2009;29:994–1001.

[6] Cheung CMG, Yeo IYS, Koh A. Photoreceptor changes in acute and resolved acute posterior multifocal placoid pigment epitheliopathy documented by spectral-domain optical coherence tomography. Arch Ophthalmol 2010;128:644–6.

[7] Goldenberg D, Habot-Wilner Z, Loewenstein A, *et al.* Spectral domain optical coherence tomography classification of acute posterior multifocal placoid pigment epitheliopathy. Retina. 2012;32(7):1403-10.

[8] Tarabishy AB, Lowder CY. Retinal pigment epithelium disturbances in acute posterior multifocal placoid pigment epitheliopathy. Eye 2010;24:1404–5.

[9] Lim WK, Buggage RR, Nussenblatt RB. Serpiginous choroiditis. Surv Ophthalmol 2005;50:231–44.

[10] Varma D, Anand S, Reddy AR, *et al.* Tuberculosis: an under-diagnosed aetiological agent in uveitis with an effective treatment. Eye 2006;20:1068–73.

[11] Punjabi OS, Rich R, Davis JL, *et al.* Imaging serpiginous choroidopathy with spectral domain optical coherence tomography. Ophthalmic Surg Lasers Imaging 2008;39:S95–98.

[12] van Velthoven MEJ, Ongkosuwito JV, Verbraak FD, *et al.* Combined en-face optical coherence tomography and confocal ophthalmoscopy findings in active multifocal and serpiginous chorioretinitis. Am J Ophthalmol 2006;141:972–5.

[13] Kedhar SR, Thorne JE, Wittenberg S, *et al.* Multifocal choroiditis with panuveitis and punctate inner choroidopathy: comparison of clinical characteristics at presentation. Retina 2007;27:1174–9.

[14] Spaide RF, Koizumi H, Freund KB. Photoreceptor outer segment abnormalities as a cause of blind spot enlargement in acute zonal occult outer retinopathy-complex diseases. Am J Ophthalmol 2008;146:111–20.

[15] Vance SK, Khan S, Klancnik JM, *et al.* Characteristic spectral-domain optical coherence tomography findings of multifocal choroiditis. Retina 2011;31:717–23.

[16] Julián K, Terrada C, Fardeau C, *et al.* Intravitreal bevacizumab as first local treatment for uveitis-related choroidal neovascularization: long-term results. Acta Ophthalmol 2011;89:179–84.

[17] Shah KH, Levinson RD, Yu F, *et al.* Birdshot chorioretinopathy. Surv Ophthalmol 2005;50:519–41.

[18] Monnet D, Levinson RD, Holland GN, *et al.* Longitudinal cohort study of patients with birdshot chorioretinopathy. III. Macular imaging at baseline. Am J Ophthalmol 2007;144:818–28.

[19] Witkin AJ, Duker JS, Ko TH, *et al.* Ultrahigh Resolution Optical Coherence Tomography of Birdshot Retinochoroidopathy. Br J Ophthalmol 2005;89:1660–1.

[20] Comander J, Loewenstein J, Sobrin L. Diagnostic testing and disease monitoring in birdshot chorioretinopathy. Semin Ophthalmol 2011;26:329–36.

[21] Krill AE, Deutman AF. Acute retinal pigment epitheliitis. Am J Ophthalmol 1972;74:193–205.

[22] Baillif S, Wolff B, Paoli V, *et al.* Retinal fluorescein and indocyanine green angiography and spectral-domain optical coherence tomography findings in acute retinal pigment epitheliitis. Retina 2011;31:1156–63.

Chapter 3

Application of Optical Coherence Tomography and Macular Holes in Ophthalmology

Robert J. Lowe and Ronald C. Gentile

Additional information is available at the end of the chapter

http://dx.doi.org/10.5772/53535

1. Introduction

Optical coherence tomography (OCT) has revolutionized how we understand macular holes. The purpose of this chapter is to describe the integration of OCT in the diagnosis, classification, and management of macular holes.

2. Definitions of macular holes

A macular hole is a full thickness defect, or hole, in the neurosensory retina located within, or just eccentric to the center of the fovea.

An impending macular hole, also known as a stage 1 macular hole, is considered the precursor to a full thickness idiopathic macular hole. Impending macular holes have a splitting of the inner retina with the clinical appearance of a foveolar cyst or pseudocyst. In some cases, this inner splitting can be associated with a defect in the underlying outer retina (Lee, Kang et al. 2011). An impending macular hole with a defect in the outer retina can have a very thin intact inner retina referred to as the roof of the impending macular hole. These impending macular holes can progress to become full thickness macular hole once a break in the inner retina or roof occurs.

Most macular holes, unless otherwise specified, refer to idiopathic macular holes. Idiopathic macular holes occur from tractional forces on the foveola at the vitreoretinal interface not associated with other causes. Other types of macular holes include those associated with trauma, high myopia, retinal detachments, lasers accidents, lightning strikes, diabetic retinopathy, and epiretinal membranes.

3. Types of macular holes

3.1. Idiopathic macular holes

Idiopathic macular holes are the most common type of macular hole. A population based chart review of patients with macular holes reported that 92% of macular holes were idiopathic. Mean age in this study was 68.6 (range 47.5–89.6) years. The prevalence of idiopathic macular holes ranges from 0.02% to 0.8%. The incidence of idiopathic macular holes was found to be 8.5 persons per 100,000 population per year (McCannel, Ensminger et al. 2009).

3.2. Traumatic macular holes

Macular holes can be associated with ocular trauma and are often referred to as traumatic macular holes. In the same population based study mentioned above, only 2% of all macular holes were traumatic macular holes (McCannel, Ensminger et al. 2009).

The formation of a traumatic macular hole is believed to be related to the rapid changes at the vitreofoveal interface that occur during the traumatic event. In a study from the Walter Reed Army Medical Center, 3% of soldiers who sustained combat related ocular trauma were found to have full thickness macular holes (Weichel and Colyer 2009). In contrast to the formation of idiopathic macular holes that may occur over the course of weeks to months, the formation of traumatic macular holes is quicker. (Johnson, McDonald et al. 2001).

Other associated findings seen in traumatic macular holes, not present in idiopathic macular holes, include retinal pigment epithelium (RPE) mottling with damaged to the RPE. Damage to the RPE appears to be directly related to the trauma. Despite the presence of RPE damage, visual recovery is still possible (Chow, Williams et al. 1999; Johnson, McDonald et al. 2001). Fortunately, the surgical closure rate (96%) and visual improvement in traumatic macular holes is similar to that found with idiopathic macular hole closure (Johnson, McDonald et al. 2001).

3.3. Myopic macular holes

Macular holes can be associated with high myopia and are referred to as myopic macular holes. High myopia is most commonly defined as a refractive error equal to or greater than −6.00 diopters of axial myopia with an axial length of greater than 26 mm (Wu and Kung 2011).

Highly myopic patients seem to be at higher risk for developing macular holes that have unique features and associations. Myopic macular holes develop as the refractive error increases (Kobayashi, Kobayashi et al. 2002) and can be associated with retinal detachments and myopic schisis. The association with retinal detachment appears greatest in the presence of a posterior staphaloma and longer axial length (greater than or equal to 30 mm).

The success rate of surgical repair of myopic macular holes is not as high as the surgical closure rate of macular holes in non-myopic eyes. Some studies have reported success rates as low at 60% and 62.5% (Patel, Loo et al. 2001; Wu and Kung 2011) compared to the 90% success rates seen in idiopathic macular hole repair. The lower success rate is believed to be related to a foreshortened retina within the staphaloma that can create residual tractional forces on the retina despite surgery (Ikuno, Sayanagi et al. 2003; Wu and Kung 2011).

3.4. Macular holes following retinal detachment surgery

Rarely, macular holes can form after retinal detachment surgery. The prevalence of macular hole formation after any type of retinal detachment surgery has been reported to be 0.9% (Benzerroug, Genevois et al. 2008). In eyes that underwent retinal detachment surgery with pars plana vitrectomy, the prevalence has ranged between 0.2% to 1.1% (Lee, Park et al. 2010; Fabian, Moisseiev et al. 2011). For reasons not well understood, macular holes forming after retinal detachment surgery tend to occur more often in macula-off retinal detachments (Benzerroug, Genevois et al. 2008). In one study, the prevalence of macular holes after retinal detachment surgery is more than 3 times greater than the prevalence of macular holes due to idiopathic causes (0.3%) (Fabian, Moisseiev et al. 2011). Fortunately, the surgical closure rate in eyes with macular holes after retinal detachment surgery is similar to the success rate of idiopathic macular hole closure, around 90% success (Benzerroug, Genevois et al. 2008; Lee, Park et al. 2010).

4. Histopathology of idiopathic macular holes

Histopathological analysis of macular holes in the 1980s helped elucidate how macular holes form. Idiopathic macular holes were found to be associated with an epiretinal membrane (ERM) leading to the wrinkling of the internal limiting membrane of the inner retina. Furthermore, cystoid macular edema within the inner nuclear and outer plexiform layers of the retina, located around these idiopathic macular holes, were also discovered. An operculum of glial cells have been found over the macular holes (Frangieh, Green et al. 1981).

From these histopathological studies, the ILM, ELM formation, and cystoid macular edema were believed to play a role in the pathogenesis of idiopathic macular holes. Many felt that vitreous traction may be implicated in the pathogenesis of macular holes, especially in cases where an operculum of glial tissue was seen on the posterior hyloid face of the vitreous (Frangieh, Green et al. 1981). Anterior-posterior traction from a posterior vitreous detachment can also convert a macular cyst to a macular hole (McDonnell, Fine et al. 1982).

At the time of these histological studies, surgical repair of macular holes was not an option. Macular holes that have closed were due to spontaneous closure. Histopathology of spontaneously closed macular holes have revealed proliferation of fibroglial cells filling and bridging the macular hole (Frangieh, Green et al. 1981). This finding may be seen in surgically closed macular holes as well.

5. Gass classification of idiopathic macular holes

Donald Gass and Robert Johnson in the late 1980s and early 1990s created a classification system for idiopathic macular holes. They divided idiopathic macular holes into 4 stages based on clinical findings using contact lens biomicroscopy. Remarkably, this was done before the clinical use of optical coherence tomography (OCT).

5.1. Stage 1

Stage 1 macular holes, also known as impending macular holes, are considered precursors of full thickness macular holes. Stage 1 macular holes are divided into 2 substages, 1A and 1B (Gass 1988). Stage 1A appears as a yellow spot in the center of the fovea (Gass 1995). The foveal yellow spot ranges between 100 to 200 μm in diameter and has flattening of the normal foveal depression (Gass 1988). Stage 1B appears as a yellow ring that measures roughly 200 to 350 μm in diameter. The yellow ring is believed to be due to the centrifugal displacement of the xanthophylls and foveal retinal tissue (Gass 1995). Visual acuity in patients with a stage 1 (impending) macular holes are usually good, but can range from 20/25 to 20/70. Retinal angiography using fluorescein dye (fluorescein angiography, or FA) of stage 1 macular holes is usually normal or may show early hyperfluorescece without late staining or leakage (Gass 1988).

5.2. Stage 2

Progression from stage 1 to a stage 2 can occur over weeks to months. Stage 2 macular holes (early hole formation) are full thickness holes of less than 400 μm in size. An early stage 2 macular hole can be located within, or just eccentric to the center of the fovea. When located centrally the holes are usually round. When the holes are located eccentric, they can be oval or crescent shaped (Gass 1995). Gass hypothesized that stage 2 macular holes start as a break located either eccentrically at one end of the yellow ring or in 2 peripheral locations. This break could enlarge along the ring and may lead to a release of an operculum of neuronal tissue into the vitreous cavity. However, if the break started centrally and enlarged, an operculum may not be found. Stage 2 macular holes are consistently hyperfluorescent early on

FA without late staining or leakage (Gass 1988). Vision is usually between 20/70 and 20/200 (Gass 1988).

5.3. Stage 3 and 4

Progression from a stage 2 to a stage 3 hole can occur over the course of several months with varying degrees of vitreofoveal separation. Stage 3 macular holes are full thickness holes of ≥ 400 μm in size without a complete posterior vitreous detachment. A stage 3 macular hole becomes a stage 4 macular hole once a complete posterior vitreous detachment occurs with detachment of the posterior vitreous hyaloid from the entire macula and optic disc (Gass 1995). Progression from a stage 3 to a stage 4 macular hole may take several years (Gass 1988). Vision usually deteriorates to about 20/200.

6. Introduction of optical coherence tomography

Optical coherence tomography (OCT) is considered the gold standard in diagnosing and classifying macular holes (Dayani, Maldonado et al. 2009). OCT scans display cross sectional, in vivo, representations of the retina. Remarkably, early histological work and Gass' clinical observations on macular holes correlate very well with what is seen on OCT. Before the advent of OCT, physicians diagnosed and characterized macular holes based on biomicroscopy and used visual acuity, amsler grid, Watzke-Allen sign, and FA testing to help confirm the diagnosis (McDonnell, Fine et al. 1982).

The advent of OCT made diagnosing macular holes easier and can distinguish macular holes from other macular pathology that, prior to OCT, was difficult. For example, OCT can differentiate macular holes from lamellar holes and pseudoholes. Also, OCT is superior to biomicoscopy in eyes with limited macular pigmentation or depigmentation. Decreased contrast between the retina, RPE and choroid (i.e. chorioretinal atrophy) when there is less pigmentation makes the biomicoscopic evaluation and diagnosis of macular holes difficult. This is especially true in the setting of high myopia and a posterior staphaloma (Coppe, Ripandelli et al. 2005; Wu and Kung 2011). In addition, the detection of an operculum has been facilitated and made more reliable with OCT. Without OCT, finding an operculum in the vitreous cavity can be difficult using biomicoscopy alone (Yuzawa, Watanabe et al. 1994).

OCTs have evolved with improvements in both resolution and acquisition times. Due to these improvements, commercially available time-domain (TD) OCT has been replaced with the newer spectral-domain (SD) OCT. Resolution of the OCT system, dependent on the bandwidth of the light source used, have increased the axial resolution of the OCT images from 10 - 20 μm in the TD OCTs to 5 - 6 μm in the SD OCTs (Sano, Shimoda et al. 2009). In addition, since SD OCTs measure the interferometric signal detected as a function of optical frequencies, it has imaging speeds 50 times faster than TD OCT and can provide a greater number of images per unit area. With SD OCT, 512 x 170 scans (horizontal x vertical) in a 6 x 6 mm^2 area can be made to ensure that all dimensions of the macular hole are not missed (Masuyama, Yamakiri et al. 2009).

7. Mechanism of macular hole formation

7.1. Idiopathic macular hole formation

Based on clinical observations, Gass proposed a mechanism of macular hole formation that involved vitreous traction on the fovea. Vitreous traction would start anteriorly from the retina and was followed by a tangential traction as the vitreous cortex above the fovea contracted (Gass 1988). The traction would create the stage 1A macular hole with continued traction causing the macular hole to progress from stage 1A to stage 4.

The high resolution imaging from OCT has lead to a better understanding of the relationship between the vitreous and retina during the formation of a macular hole. Using OCT the pathophysiology of a macular hole can be divided into three phases and one pivotal event. The first phase, or formation phase, is the initiating event. The first phase is followed by the pivotal event that determines if the macular hole enters the second phase, or the progression phase. The third phase, or closure phase, most often occurs surgically. In some cases, the closure phase can occur spontaneously.

Anterior –posterior contraction of the cortical vitreous from the fovea in time-lapsed OCT morphing videos appears to be the initiating event, or phase 1, in idiopathic macular hole formation. In phase 1 the anterior-posterior traction comes from the detachment of the posterior hyloid from the fovea. The anterior-posterior traction may cause a break in the ILM and/or ELM. If a break occurs in both the ILM and ELM, the foveal integrity can become destabilized, and the pivotal event occurs.

After the pivotal event, fluid may enter the breaks in the ILM and ELM and cause hydration of the neurosensory retina with cystic formation at the edges of the macular hole. This accumulation of cystic fluid, or phase 2, leads to progression and enlargement of the macular hole. This cystic hydration leads to further elevation of the edges of the macular hole off the RPE with progressive enlargement of the macular hole. In phase 3, or closure phase, migration of glial cells over the macular hole leads to closure of the macular hole and subsequent reabsorb the cystic and subretinal fluid by the RPE pump (Gentile, Landa et al. 2010).

7.2. Traumatic macular hole formation

It was hypothesized that formation of traumatic macular holes occur when the blunt ocular trauma causes a rapid compression of the cornea and expansion of the globe. This force leads to expansion of the equator, flattening of the posterior pole, and subsequent posterior expansion of the posterior pole. The tractional force on the thin fovea is thought to lead to the formation of a macular hole (Johnson, McDonald et al. 2001). This mechanism can occur without a posterior vitreous detachment. OCT of traumatic macular holes have shown a full thickness macular hole without a posterior vitreous detachment in patients who report immediate vision loss after the trauma (Yamashita, Uemara et al. 2002). If there is a delay in vision loss and a delay in the formation of the macular hole after trauma, this might occur if there is persistent vitreous adhesion to the fovea after the

http://dx.doi.org/10.5772/53535

trauma. The persistent vitreous adhesion, as demonstrated on OCT, can cause traction on the fovea and lead to delayed dehiscence with later onset of vision loss. Once the persistent vitreous adhesion resolves, traumatic macular holes have been shown to spontaneously close (Yamashita, Uemara et al. 2002).

7.3. Macular hole formation in high myopia

OCT has been utilized to helped understand how macular holes form in highly myopic eyes. Macular hole formation in highly myopic eyes can arise from macular retinoschisis (Sun, Liu et al. 2010). Retinoschisis is a splitting of the retinal layers and was first described in highly myopic eyes with posterior staphalomas using OCT (Takano and Kishi 1999). It is hypothesized that macular holes develop in highly myopic eyes from macular retinoschisis and overlying vitreofoveal traction (Benhamou, Massin et al. 2002; Shimada, Ohno-Matsui et al. 2006; Sun, Liu et al. 2010). Two patterns of macular hole formation from myopic macular retinoschisis have been described and are differentiated by the location of the initial lamellar defect. Pattern 1 starts with an outer retinal lamellar defect that unroofs and leads to a full thickness macular hole. Pattern 2 starts with an inner retinal lamellar defect with the defect progressing posteriorly to the RPE to become a full thickness macular hole. Time to progression of pattern 1 and 2 to become a full thickness macular hole can be 11 and 9 months, respectively (Sun, Liu et al. 2010).

7.4. Macular hole formation after pars plana vitrectomy

The mechanism of macular hole formation after pars plana vitrectomy is unclear. This poses interesting challenges to the belief that the inciting mechanism of idiopathic macular hole formation is from anterior-posterior vitreous traction. Vitreous traction is not present in these eyes because they have already undergone vitrectomy and in most cases a posterior vitreous detachment has already occurred.

Furthermore, macular holes seen after retinal detachment repair tend to occur in macula-off retinal detachments. It is unclear if having subretinal fluid under the fovea plays a role in macular hole formation in these cases (Benzerroug, Genevois et al. 2008).

Various mechanisms have been proposed to help explain how macular holes form after pars plana vitrectomy for retinal detachment repair. These mechanisms include traction during the surgical repair or traction from the ILM, ERM or residual vitreous cortex (Fabian, Moisseiev et al. 2011).

7.5. Formation of aborted macular holes

In addition to fully understanding how macular holes develop, it is also important to visualize how macular holes can abort. The mechanism of aborted macular holes depends on the occurrence of a posterior vitreous foveal detachment during stage 1 of the macular hole. If the posterior vitreous detaches from the fovea after formation of a stage 1 macular hole, progression to stage 2 macular hole is aborted about 50% of the time (Gass 1995).

In these cases, there may be improvement or stabilization of visual acuity to 20/30 or better. Clinically there is also improvement in the yellow ring seen on biomicroscopy, and in some cases resolution of the early hyperfluorescece seen on FA (Gass 1988). However, despite resolution of the foveal elevation seen in stage 1, a lamellar defect of the inner retinal layers can still occur. In these cases, an operculum over a lamellar defect or a vitreous opacity overlying a normal fovea may be present in 1/3 of cases (Johnson and Gass 1988; Gass 1995).

8. Optical coherence tomography characterization of stage 1 through 4 macular holes

8.1. Stage 1A

The use of OCT has given us an in vivo visualization of macular holes that we could never have achieved clinically. New descriptions of findings have been characterized based on OCT. For example, stage 1A macular holes were found to have a triangular detachment of the foveola on OCT. The mean width of the foveolar detachment was further characterized as 167.7 μm with a range between 146 and 205 μm. The triangular detachment of the foveola was felt to be a detachment of the posterior tips of the cone outer segments (COST) (Takahashi, Nagaoka et al. 2011).

The COST and its relationship to macular holes were further described using OCT. The anterior-posterior vitreal traction onto the fovea may extend through the Müller cells of the retina onto the photoreceptors to cause a localized photoreceptor detachment or COST detachment (Takahashi, Nagaoka et al. 2010). The COST detachment can enlarge horizontally and anteriorly to involve the inner segment/outer segment junction (Takahashi, Nagaoka et al. 2011).

After complete posterior vitreous detachment, a stage 1A macular hole can abort and become an aborted macular hole. The triangular detachment of the COST and yellow spot may resolve. Also in some cases a residual defect in the outer retina, specifically the junction between the inner segments and outer segments, can be seen underneath the fovea in the aborted macular holes (Takahashi, Nagaoka et al. 2011).

8.2. Stage 1B

Stage 1B (Figures 1 and 2) macular holes, compared to Stage 1A macular holes, were found to involve both the inner and outer retinal layers of the fovea (Takahashi, Nagaoka et al. 2011). The roof or inner layer of the stage 1B macular hole remains intact, and the outer layer develops a break with the RPE layer becoming devoid of photoreceptors (Takahashi, Nagaoka et al. 2011). A portion of the detached outer retina consisting of cone photoreceptors may even become part of the roof of the macular hole (Takahashi, Nagaoka et al. 2010).

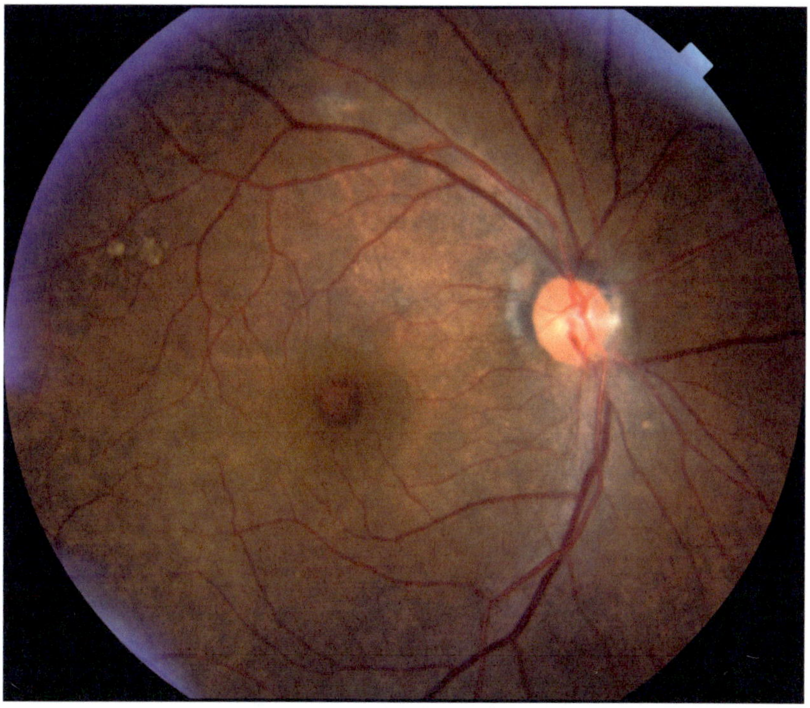

Figure 1. Fundus photo of a stage 1B macular hole

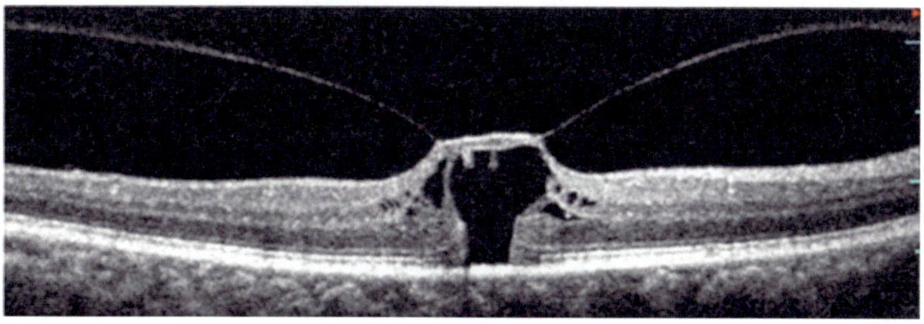

*All OCT images in the book chapter were obtained using the Cirrus HD-OCT Model 4000, Carl Zeiss Meditec, Inc. or Spectral OCT SLO, Opko/OTI, Inc.

Figure 2. OCT* of the same eye from figure 1 showing a stage 1B macular hole. There is a defect in the outer layers of the retina.

8.3. Stage 2

OCT can show a break in the roof of a stage 2 full thickness macular hole (Figure 3). The patient, a 69 year old woman, had a decrease in visual acuity (VA) to 20/100 (Figure 3). After a pars plana vitrectomy (PPV), ILM peel, gas tamponade and eventual cataract surgery, vision improved to 20/20.

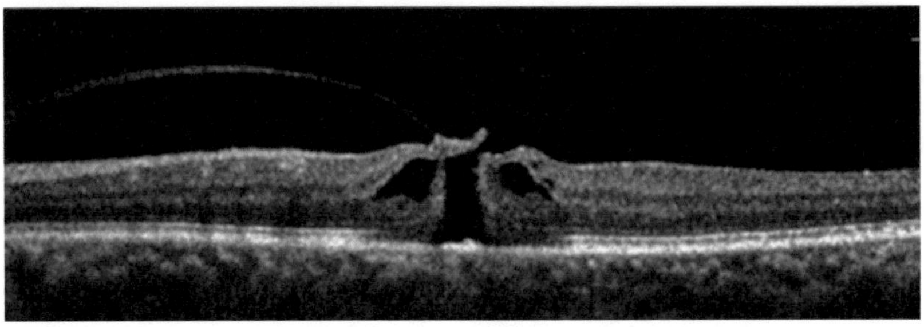

Figure 3. OCT of a stage 2 macular hole with a break in the roof and cystoid hydration.

8.4. Stage 3

OCT can show a full thickness macular hole with an operculum. Figure 4, a 70 year old woman, with a VA of Finger Count had surgical repair of the macular hole and subsequent cataract surgery. VA improved to 20/40, 1 year after her primary surgery.

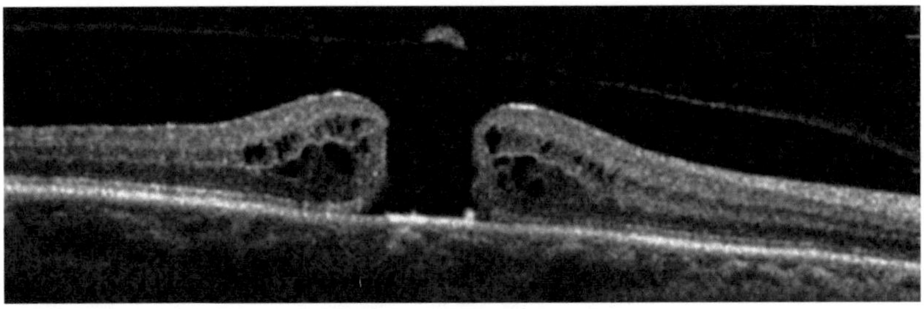

Figure 4. Full thickness stage 3 macular hole with overlying operculum. This macular hole would be classified as stage 4 if the posterior vitreous completely detached from the macula and optic nerve.

9. Surgical repair of macular holes

In 1991, Kelly and Wendel reported on the surgical management of macular holes. This involved a pars plana vitrectomy, creation of a posterior vitreous detachment if one was not already present, removal of an ERM if present, gas tamponade, and face down positioning. Initial anatomical success rates were reported to be 58% with improvement in visual acuity (Kelly and Wendel 1991). Success rates improved to 73% in a later report by the same group. Overall, greater success of anatomical closure was found in smaller macular holes with symptoms that were less than 6 months in duration (Wendel, Patel et al. 1993).

9.1. Internal limiting membrane peeling during surgical repair

Following Kelly and Wendel's initial report, peeling the ILM layer of the innermost portion of the retina was published. In 1999, Park et. al. described a case series of 58 eyes who underwent an ERM peel or ILM peel if an ERM was not present. A 91% anatomical success rate was reported. They suggested that removing the ILM aided in relieving tangential traction. This traction may come from contractile myofibroblastic cells that proliferate over the ILM (Park, Sipperley et al. 1999).

In order to remove traction from the myofibroblastic cells over the ILM, the ILM must also be removed during macular hole surgery. Furthermore, it is thought that contraction from the ILM displaces photoreceptors that may lead to enlargement of the macular hole. Once the ILM is surgically removed, the photoreceptors may be able to return towards the center of the hole and promote macular hole closure (Sano, Shimoda et al. 2009).

In a comparison of macular hole repair with and without ILM peeling, an anatomical success rate of 100% (116/116 eyes) with ILM peeling vs 82% success rate (36/44 eyes) without ILM peeling was reported. However, in the cases without ILM peeling, an ERM if present was not removed. The remaining ERM may have adversely affected the closure rate in these patients (Brooks 2000).

In a randomized clinical control trial performed in the United Kingdom, patients with idiopathic stage 2 or 3 macular holes were randomized to ILM peeling vs no ILM peeling. In the ILM peeling group, the ILM was stained with 0.15% trypan blue to aid in the visualization of the transparent ILM. The rate of macular hole closure in the ILM peeling group vs no ILM peeling at 1 month was 84% and 48%, respectively. The rate of macular hole reoperation in the ILM peeling group vs no ILM peeling by 6 months was 12% and 48%, respectively. At the conclusion of the study, the authors recommended ILM peeling in the repair of macular holes. ILM peeling was felt to be safe and more cost effective, with a higher success rate for macular hole closure (Lois, Burr et al. 2011).

9.2. The use of intraoperative optical coherence tomography

OCT has been used as an adjuctive tool in the operating room. It has helped shed light on the change in the contour of macular holes before and after ILM peeling. OCT before and after ILM peeling at the edge of the macular hole in one patient documented the relaxation and elevation of the edge of the macular hole that was thought to aid in the surgical repair of the macular hole. After removal of the ILM, the base diameter of the macular holes decreased while the height increased (Dayani, Maldonado et al. 2009). Intraoperative OCT also demonstrated a decrease in macular hole base diameter immediately after air-fluid exchange. Macular hole closure was even seen intraoperatively in a stage 3 macular hole and in a traumatic macular hole during the air-fluid exchange (Hayashi, Yagou et al. 2011).

9.3. The use of optical coherence tomography in gas filled eyes

Recently, there have been reports of imaging macular holes after repair in gas filled eyes. This was difficult before the advent of the newer generation SD OCT. Before SD OCT, the older TD OCTs were unable to image eyes under gas tamponade due to the excessive light reflectivity of the gas-retinal interface and difficulty in imaging the correct area, easily missed with TD OCT (Masuyama, Yamakiri et al. 2009).

Imaging the macular hole area is accomplished more easily using SD OCT. SD OCT can quickly perform serial scans over the macular area. Using SD OCT, it was found that imaging though gas was easier with a complete gas fill. Once the gas level decreased to a 70% fill, the light reflex from the lower meniscus of the gas made imaging of the macular hole more difficult. Imaging became possible again once the gas fill reached 50% (Masuyama, Yamakiri et al. 2009).

A recent study examining how quickly macular holes can close postoperatively using OCT found closed macular holes in 10 of 13 eyes (76.9%) on postoperative day 1 and an additional 2 eyes that closed by postoperative day 2 (Masuyama, Yamakiri et al. 2009). Sano et. al. had similar experiences with SD OCT imaging of macular holes through gas. Of the over 90% of eyes they were able to image on postoperative day 1, over 90% were found to be closed (Sano, Inoue et al. 2011).

After the vitrectomy and ILM peeling for the surgical repair of macular holes, patients were instructed to remain in a face down position so that the gas will be juxtaposed against the macular hole. The use of SD OCT in the immediate postoperative period may help in limiting the amount of face down positioning needed. Patients may consider stopping their face down positioning once the macular hole appears closed on OCT, which may be as early as postoperative day 1 (Masuyama, Yamakiri et al. 2009; Sano, Inoue et al. 2011).

9.4. Silicone oil tamponade

For some patients, face down positioning may be impossible. In such patients, silicone oil tamponade can be a viable option. Oster et. al. demonstrated using SD OCT that there was no difference in silicone oil tamponade with face forward or face down positioning in 75% of the study eyes (Oster, Mojana et al. 2010).

The use of silicone oil for myopic macular hole repair without face down positioning has been show to be successful in the closure of myopic macular holes with subsequent improvement of vision. Myopic macular holes were successfully closed in 22 of 24 eyes (92%) using silicone oil after ILM peeling. These eyes had an average axial length of 29.6 ± 1.8 mm and an average of 23.3 ± 14.0 months of tamponade (Nishimura, Kimura et al. 2011).

Furthermore, Jumper et. al. found similar OCT findings of early post-surgical macular hole closure through silicone oil tamponade as compared to gas tamponade. As early as the first postoperative day in eyes with silicone oil tamponade, flattening of the edges of the macular hole has been shown using OCT. This flattening of the edges was accompanied by a decrease in both the size of the intraretinal cystic spaces and in the subretinal fluid located at the cuff of the macular hole (Jumper, Gallemore et al. 2000).

However, Oster et. al. has demonstrated that silicone oil tamponade may have some limitations when compared with gas tamonade. Supine positioning may cause the silicone oil to rise anteriorly and a fluid pocket to form between the macular hole and silicone oil interface. In 7 of 10 eyes, the silicone oil bridged the macular hole while in the remaining 3 eyes, the silicone oil filled the macular hole and was in contact with the RPE. If the silicone oil fills the macular hole, it may prevent the complete close of the macular hole. Furthermore, silicone oil contact with the RPE may be toxic to the subfoveal RPE. This potential damage to the RPE does not occur with gas tamponade (Oster, Mojana et al. 2010).

10. Two OCT classifications to define macular hole closure

OCT has helps characterize macular hole closure. Two groups have described their own classification for macular hole closures.

Kang et. al. described macular hole closure as either type 1 or type 2 as imaged on OCT. Type 1 closure is defined as the presence of a continuous layer of retinal tissue bridging the macular hole. Normal foveal contour is seen in type 1 macular hole closures. Type 2 closure is defined as an interruption of retinal tissue between the edges of the macular hole. On OCT, the edges of the macular hole were attached to the underlying RPE without subretinal fluid. According to Kang et al. type 1 and 2 closures represent successful anatomical closure of macular holes (Kang, Ahn et al. 2003). As expected, type 1 closure was associated with better visual outcomes than type 2 closure. Larger macular holes (mean diameter: 674 μm) were associated with type 2 closures, while smaller holes (mean diameter: 469 μm) were more associated with type 1 closures (Kang, Ahn et al. 2003).

Tornambe et. al. provided a similar OCT classification system divided also into type 1 and type 2 macular hole closures. Type 1 represented a flat and closed macular hole configuration. Type 2 closure is an open macular hole with flat edges. Both types were considered successful macular hole closure. In comparison, a failed macular hole closure was seen as an open macular hole with the edges being elevated by the subretinal fluid underneath (Tornambe, Poliner et al. 1998).

11. Cases of surgical repair of macular holes

11.1. Idiopathic macular hole

A 69 year old woman presented with an idiopathic macular hole. The macular hole was stage 2 with a break in the overlying roof with cystoid hydration at the edges of the macular hole (Figure 5). Visual acuity was Finger Count. The patient underwent a PPV, indocyanine green (ICG) staining of the ILM, ILM peeling and gas tamponade. After face down positioning, the macular hole closed (Figure 6). After subsequent cataract surgery, 6 months after initial macular hole surgical repair, vision improved to 20/60.

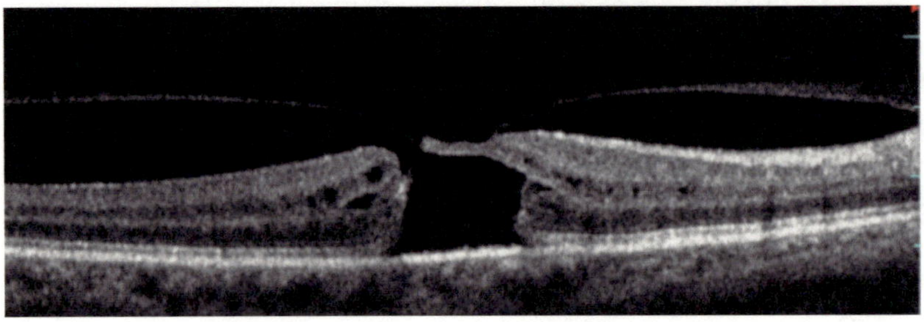

Figure 5. Preoperative OCT of an eccentric stage 2 macular hole with vitreous adhesion to the roof of the macular hole

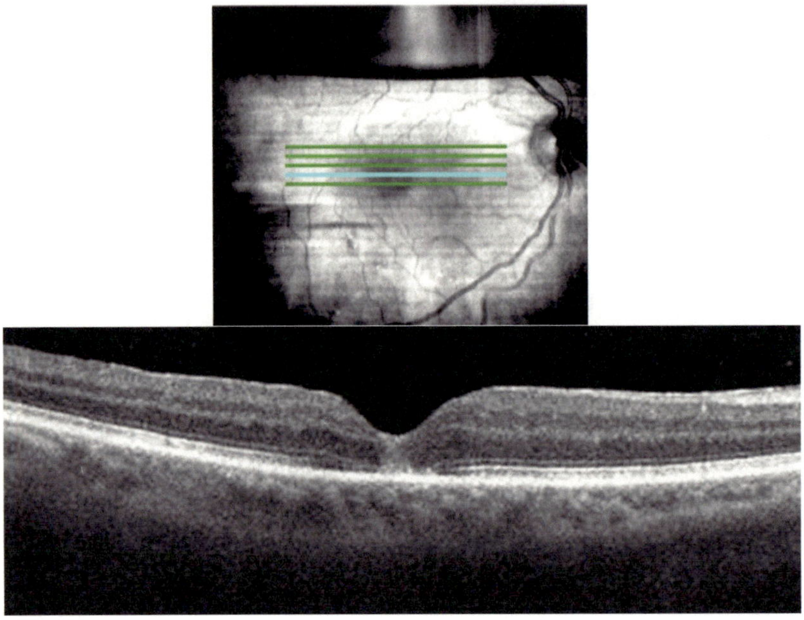

Figure 6. Postoperative OCT of the closed macular hole one month after surgical repair. Note the residual gas bubble obscuring view of the superior retinal blood vessels at the top photo.

11.2. Traumatic macular hole

A 31 year old man presented with a traumatic macular hole following an airbag injury (Figure 7). Vision initially was 20/100 with OCT (Figure 8) revealing a full thickness macular hole with subretinal hemorrhage. There was an associated choroidal rupture (Figure 9). Despite no change in visual acuity, repeat OCT two weeks later revealed progressive cystoid hydration at the edges of the macular hole with subretinal fluid (Figure 10). The patient underwent repair of the macular hole with PPV, ILM peeling, and gas tamponade with closure of the macular hole (Figure 11) and improvement in vision to 20/30.

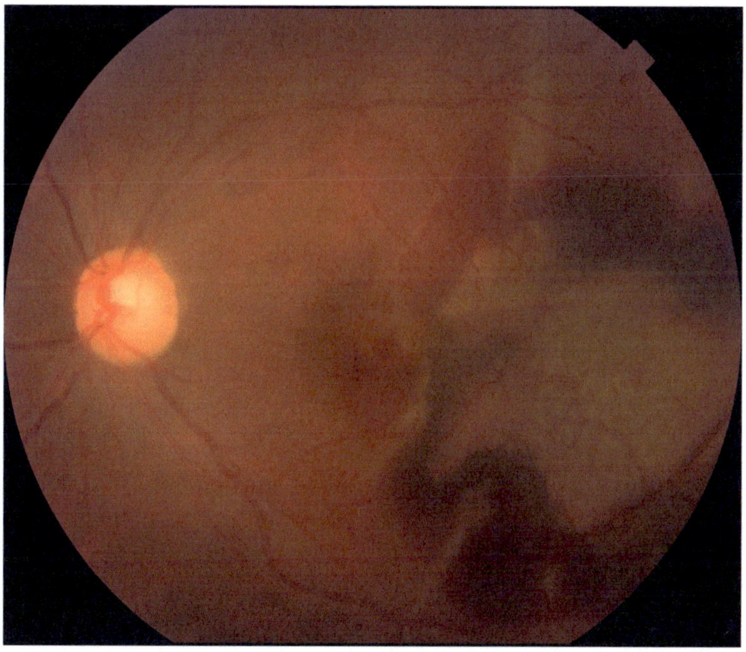

Figure 7. Fundus photo of the traumatic macular hole with associated subretinal hemorrhage and choroidal rupture

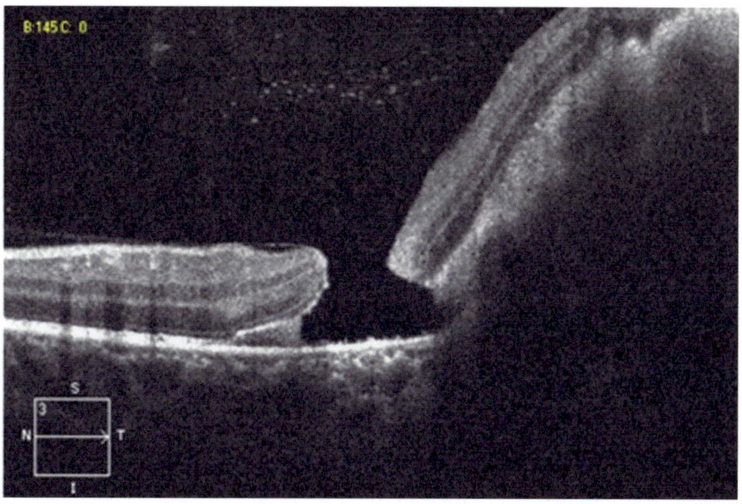

Figure 8. OCT of the traumatic macular hole and subretinal hemorrhage

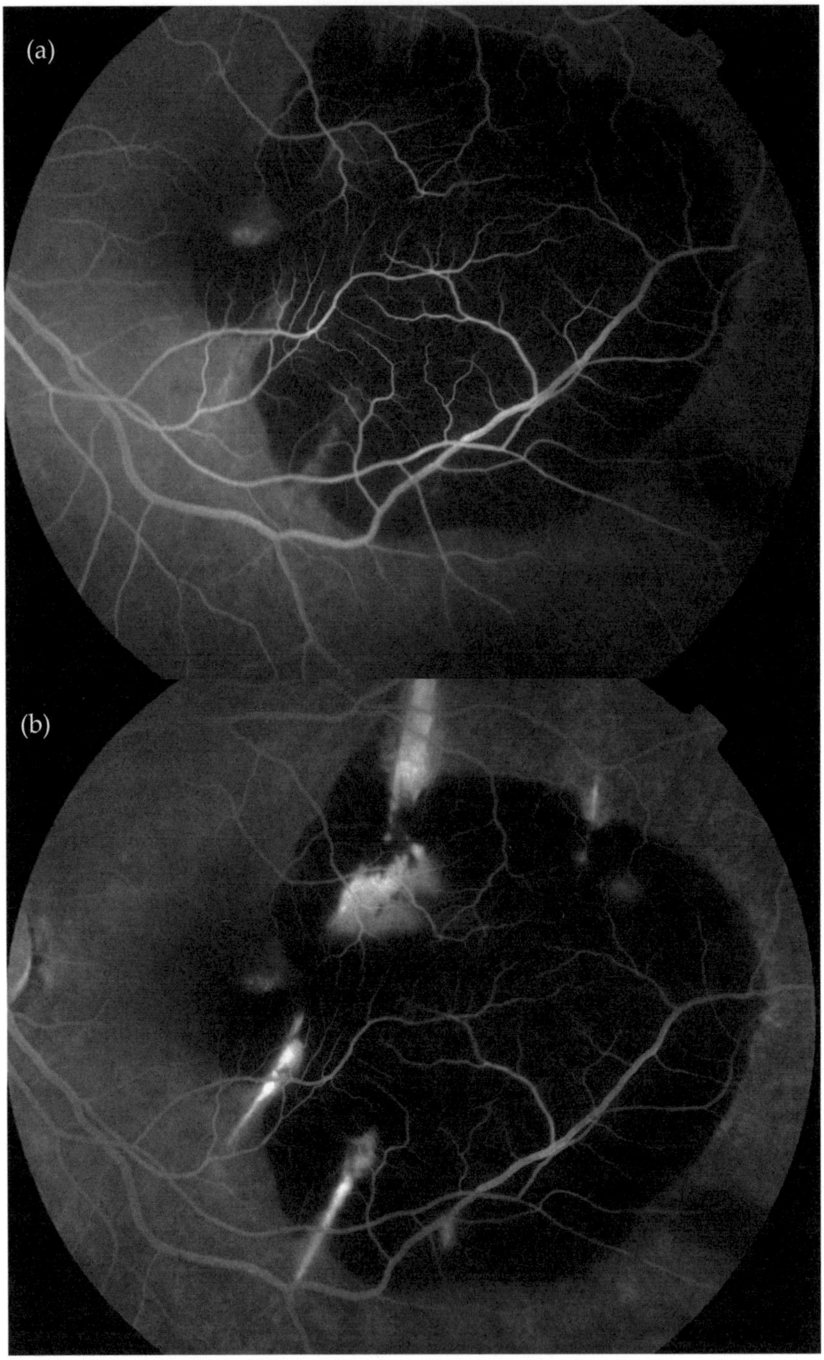

Figure 9. FA of an early and late frame showing the initial hyperflourescence of the macular hole (a) with an increase in hyperfluoresence of the choroidal rupture (b). The area of decreased fluorescence corresponds to the subretinal hemorrhage.

http://dx.doi.org/10.5772/53535

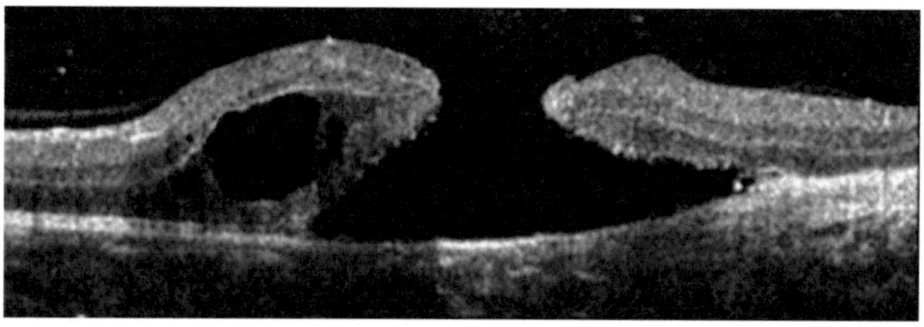

Figure 10. OCT showing enlargement of the macular hole with subretinal fluid and cystic hydration

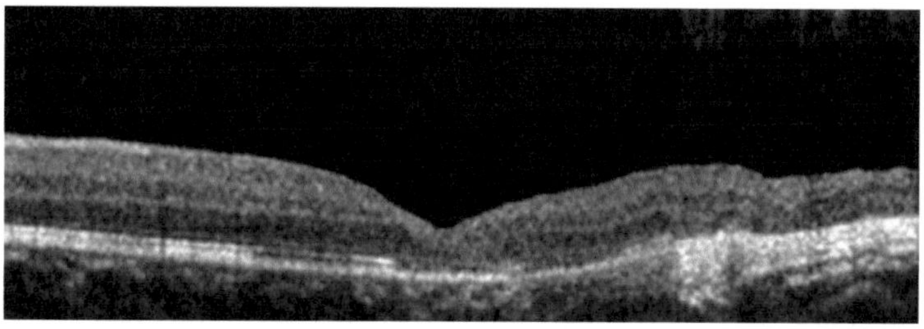

Figure 11. OCT showing closure of the macular hole and improvement of the vision after PPV, ILM peel, and gas tamponade

11.3. High myopic macular hole and retinal detachment

Retinal detachment repair from a macular hole in an eye with high myopia can be challenging. A 68 year old, highly myopic women presented with a macular hole and retinal detachment. Vision was Finger Count. Her fellow eye had myopic macular retinoschisis (Figure 12). She underwent a PPV and ILM peel with silicone oil tamponade to repair her retinal detachment and macular hole. Two weeks after retinal detachment repair, the vision improved to 20/150 (Figure 13). One month after retinal detachment repair, she subsequently underwent removal of the silicone oil with additional ILM peel and gas tamponade to repair the macular hole. Two weeks after macular hole repair, her OCT revealed a closed/flat macular hole configuration (Figure 14). Six months after macular hole repair, the visual acuity was 20/100.

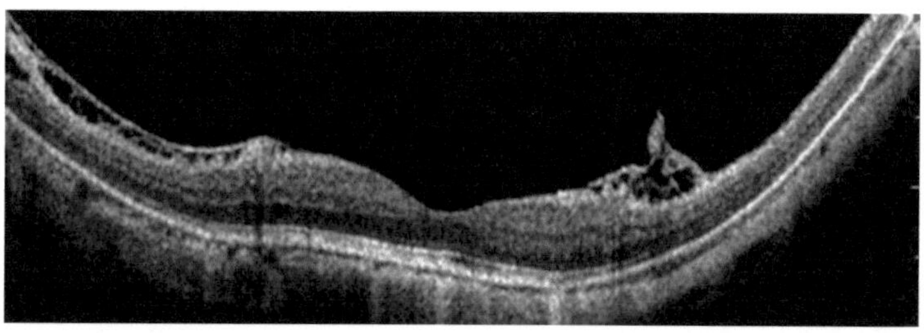

Figure 12. Myopic retinoschisis in the fellow eye

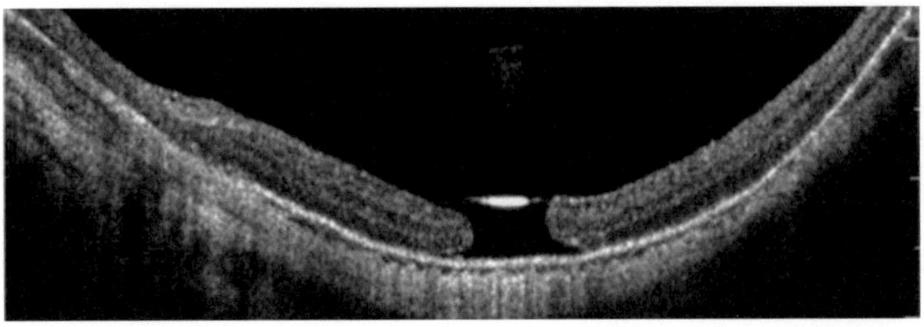

Figure 13. OCT showing an open macular hole after retinal detachment repair with membrane peel and silicone oil tamponade. Note the high reflective layer of the edge of the silicone oil tamponade over the macular hole.

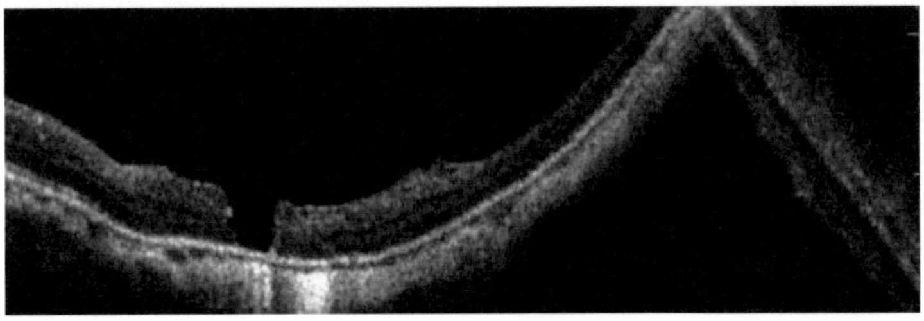

Figure 14. OCT of a flat and closed macular hole closure configuration after macular hole repair.

11.4. Macular hole formation after retinal detachment repair

A macular hole can occur after retinal detachment repair. A 60 year old patient presented with a macula involving retinal detachment and a visual acuity of Finger Count. Three weeks after retinal detachment repair, central vision did not improve and a macular hole was present (Figure 15). Subsequently, the patient underwent ICG staining, ILM peeling, and gas tamponade (Figure 16 and 17). Visual acuity improved to 20/400 six months after macular hole closure.

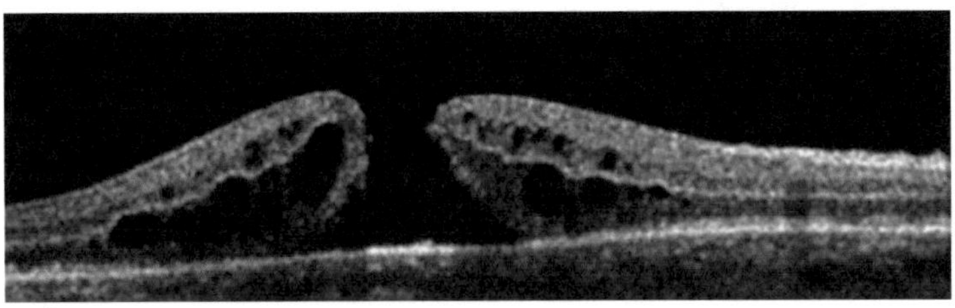

Figure 15. Macular hole formed after retinal detachment repair.

http://dx.doi.org/10.5772/53535

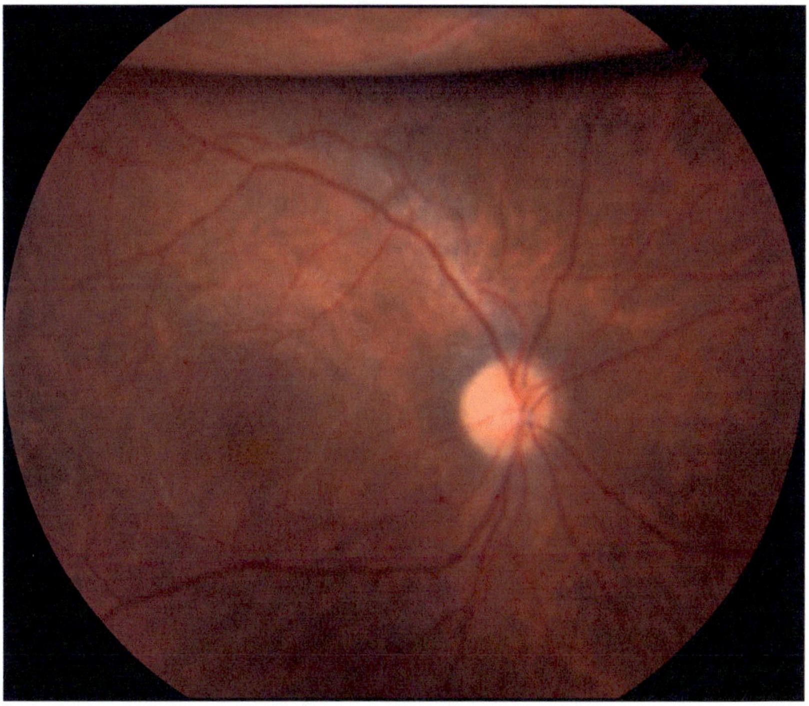

Figure 16. One month after macular hole repair: Fundus photograph showing an area of the macula devoid of ILM after ILM peel with residual superior gas bubble

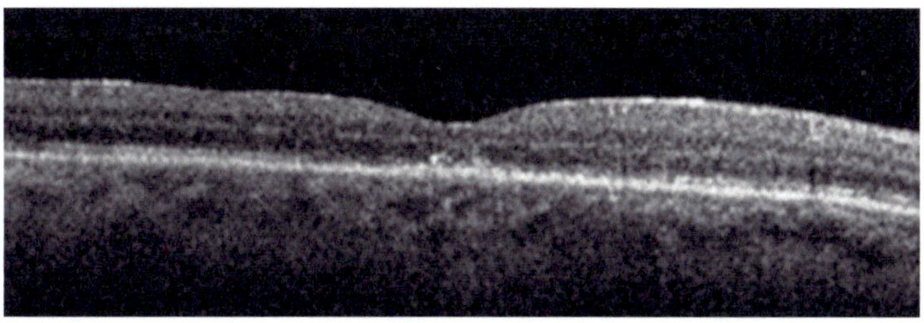

Figure 17. One month after macular hole repair: OCT showing a closed macular hole after ILM peel and gas tamponade

12. Mechanism of macular hole closure

12.1. Postsurgical macular hole closure

The mechanism of macular hole closure is better understood with the aid of OCT. Masuyama et. al. proposed that the formation of a bridge of tissue over the hole begins the macular hole closure. Neural tissue bridges the macular hole after the removal of the internal limiting membrane and during the interaction of the hole with the gas tamponade. After bridge formation, a seal is created and the subretinal and intraretinal fluid is reabsorbed to close the macular hole (Masuyama, Yamakiri et al. 2009). This subsequent reabsorption of the cystic edema and then subretinal fluid leads to the return of the foveal contour (Gentile, Landa et al. 2010). Until the gliotic wound matures, this neural tissue bridge may be unstable (Masuyama, Yamakiri et al. 2009) and the macular hole can reopen (Takahashi and Kishi 2000). Wound healing may continue though the formation of a mature gliotic plug that joins the two ends of the bridge to seal the hole. The gliotic plug that forms to close the macular hole has also been documented on histopathology (Funata, Wendel et al. 1992).

12.2. Spontaneous macular hole closure

12.2.1. Spontaneous idiopathic macular hole closure

In an observational case series of 97 eyes, Yuzawa, et. al. reported 6% of study eyes experienced a spontaneous resolution of their macular hole with improvement of their vision from 20/100 - 20/200 to 20/20 - 20/60. This occurred after an average of 25 months (range, 7 to 41 months). Better visual outcomes were seen if reattachment occurred before 24 months. Reasons attributed to the disappearance of the macular hole included the contraction of an epiretinal membrane over the macular hole, fibroglial tissue growth, retinal pigment epithelial hyperplasia over the hole, and reattachment of the operculum after posterior vitreous detachment (Yuzawa, Watanabe et al. 1994).

A subsequent observation of spontaneous macular hole closure using OCT was reported by Takahashi et. al. They proposed a mechanism of spontaneous macular hole closure that was similar to surgical macular hole closure. Macular hole closure occurred spontaneously after resolution of vitreal-foveal traction. The formation of a bridge of retinal tissue that emerged from the edge of the macular hole extended centrally over 3 to 6 weeks and closed the hole. After formation of the bridge, the subfoveal and intraretinal cystic fluid was absorbed by the RPE pump by 8 months (Takahashi and Kishi 1999).

12.2.2. Spontaneous traumatic macular hole closure

OCT has also been used to formulate a possible mechanism for spontaneous traumatic macular hole closure. Spontaneous closure of traumatic macular holes has been reported to occur between 3 to 6 months after the trauma. These cases were in young patients ranging from 11 to 19 years of age in macular holes that were less than 1/3 disc diameter in size without any cuff of subretinal fluid. The mechanism of hole closure was thought to be proliferation of glial and RPE cells at the edges of the hole (Yamada, Sakai et al. 2002). Another series of 18 patients with traumatic macular holes were followed by Yamashita et al. Eight patients (44%), age ranging from 11 to 21 years, had spontaneous closure of the macular hole. These cases also involved smaller macular holes of less then 1/3 disc diameters in size. Holes had closed between 1 week to 4 months after the trauma with improvement in visual acuity (Yamashita, Uemara et al. 2002). The mechanism of bridging tissue seen after surgical repair has also been documented in spontaneous traumatic macular hole closure (Menchini, Virgili et al. 2003).

13. Morphological changes after macular hole closure

OCT imaging of surgically closed macular holes has been showed to aid in predicting visual outcome. The preservation of the external limiting membrane (ELM) layer and photoreceptor inner and outer segment (IS/OS) junction seems to predict visual acuity and photoreceptor cell survival (Shimozono, Oishi et al. 2011). This is believed to be because the ELM represents the junction between the Müller cells and photoreceptor cells (Bottoni, De Angelis et al. 2011) and the IS/OS junction represents the integrity of photoreceptor alignment. Furthermore, the outer foveal thickness measured between the ELM and inner layer of the RPE may be a surrogate to outer segment regeneration (Shimozono, Oishi et al. 2011). An increase in outer foveal thickness 6 months after surgery is associated with better visual outcomes. In addition, ELM and IS/OS defects are associated with worse visual acuity after macular hole surgical repair (Shimozono, Oishi et al. 2011).

Visual recovery after macular hole closure is thought to occur after the detached photoreceptors at the edges of the macular hole reattach to the RPE (Yuzawa, Watanabe et al. 1994). Overall, vision improves when the outer segments elongate (increase in outer foveal thickness) with subsequent realignment of the photoreceptors (return of the IS/OS junction) as seen on OCT. An intact ELM (viable photoreceptor cells) needs to be present before the process of visual recovery begins (Shimozono, Oishi et al. 2011). After macular hole closure, the ELM appears before the IS/OS layer returns. In a study by Bottoni, et. al., there were no cases seen where there was a continuous IS/OS junction and a discontinuous ELM after macular hole closure (Bottoni, De Angelis et al. 2011). Early disruption of the ELM during the postoperative period may be indicative of a poor visual outcome (Shimozono, Oishi et al. 2011).

Despite the successful reapproximation of the photoreceptors during macular hole closure, the status of the IS/OS layer on OCT can still vary (Sano, Shimoda et al. 2009). When comparing the continuity or discontinuity of the IS/OS layer, a continuous IS/OS in the fovea was associated with better visual outcomes at 6 months. A discontinuous IS/OS layer appears to represent damaged and/or missing photoreceptor outer segments (Sano, Shimoda et al. 2009).

14. Masquerades and differential diagnosis

OCT has helped in differentiating macular holes from clinically similar diagnoses. Making the correct diagnosis is important and will determine the medical and surgical management of these conditions.

Pseudoholes from an ERM and lamellar holes may be difficult to distinguish from full thickness macular holes without the aid of OCT. On OCT, an overlying contracted epiretinal membrane may show the vertical edges of a pseudohole with the neurosensory retina still intact above the RPE. Pseudoholes from an ERM (Figure 18) are more likely to have normal central foveal thickness with thickened perifoveal retina compared to lamellar holes that usually have a thinner and irregular center with normal perifoval thickness (Haouchine, Massin et al. 2004).

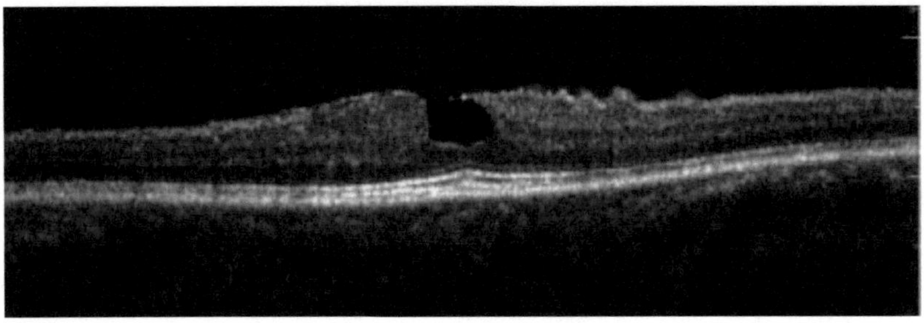

Figure 18. 60 year old woman with an ERM and pseudohole and 20/50 vision.

Lamellar macular holes are not true holes. Instead, they consist of defects in the inner retina with varying degrees of foveal thinning (Yeh, Chen et al. 2010). OCT has greatly enhanced our ability to diagnose lamellar holes, especially in highly myopic eyes. (Tanaka, Shimada et al. 2011). Findings on OCT include a discontinuous inner retinal layer, splitting of the inner retinal layer, and an irregular foveal contour. Lamellar macular holes are believed in some cases to be the result of aborted macular holes. Inner retinal defects may be due to the rupture and subsequent loss of the roof of an inner cyst of a stage 1 macular hole (Yeh, Chen et al. 2010).

However, lamellar macular holes progressing to full thickness holes have occurred (Takahashi and Kishi 2000; Tanaka, Shimada et al. 2011). These lamellar macular holes tend to have a horizontal split between the inner and outer retina that emanate from the center (Haouchine, Massin et al. 2004).

In addition, OCT can quantify the extent of vitreofoveal traction and differentiate vitreomacular traction syndrome from stage 1A or stage 1B macular holes. Vitreomacular traction syndromes have a much broader based of vitreal-retinal adhesions compared to the focal areas of vitreal-foveal adhesions seen in stage 1A or 1B macular holes (Comander, Gardiner et al. 2011). Furthermore, OCT has helped in differentiating the yellow spot seen on biomicroscopy in stage 1A macular holes from the yellow spots seen in central serous chroidopathy, ERM, or vitelliform dystrophy (Gass 1995).

Solar retinopathy can also have an appearance similar to a small full thickness macular hole. When solar retinopathy initially presents after solar exposure, it has the appearance of a yellow spot similar to what is seen in a stage 1A macular hole. Late findings in solar retinopathy involve a rectangular shaped outer retinal defect with straight edges that encompass an area from the RPE to the external limiting membrane. This outer retinal defect may be difficult to distinguish from a closed macular hole with a persistent similarly shaped outer retinal defect (Comander, Gardiner et al. 2011).

15. Conclusion

Our understanding of macular holes has come a long way from the initial descriptions by Gass to our current imaging with OCT. OCT has provided an in vivo ability to see changes in the retina that we were not able to obtain without histopathology. Correlating clinical findings, understanding the mechanism of macular hole formation and closure, and differentiating masquerades have been made possible with the aid of OCT technology.

Author details

Robert J. Lowe[1,2] and Ronald C. Gentile[1]

1 The New York Eye and Ear Infirmary, New York, USA and New York Medical College, Valhalla, NY, USA

2 Kaiser Permanente Medical Group, Walnut Creek, California, USA

References

[1] Benhamou, N., P. Massin, et al. (2002). "Macular retinoschisis in highly myopic eyes." Am J Ophthalmol 133(6): 794-800.

[2] Benzerroug, M., O. Genevois, et al. (2008). "Results of surgery on macular holes that develop after rhegmatogenous retinal detachment." Br J Ophthalmol 92(2): 217-219.

[3] Bottoni, F., S. De Angelis, et al. (2011). "The dynamic healing process of idiopathic macular holes after surgical repair: a spectral-domain optical coherence tomography study." Invest Ophthalmol Vis Sci 52(7): 4439-4446.

[4] Brooks, H. L., Jr. (2000). "Macular hole surgery with and without internal limiting membrane peeling." Ophthalmology 107(10): 1939-1948; discussion 1948-1939.

[5] Chow, D. R., G. A. Williams, et al. (1999). "Successful closure of traumatic macular holes." Retina 19(5): 405-409.

[6] Comander, J., M. Gardiner, et al. (2011). "High-Resolution Optical Coherence Tomography Findings in Solar Maculopathy and the Differential Diagnosis of Outer Retinal Holes." Am J Ophthalmol.

[7] Coppe, A. M., G. Ripandelli, et al. (2005). "Prevalence of asymptomatic macular holes in highly myopic eyes." Ophthalmology 112(12): 2103-2109.

[8] Dayani, P. N., R. Maldonado, et al. (2009). "Intraoperative use of handheld spectral domain optical coherence tomography imaging in macular surgery." Retina 29(10): 1457-1468.

[9] Fabian, I. D., E. Moisseiev, et al. (2011). "Macular Hole After Vitrectomy for Primary Rhegmatogenous Retinal Detachment." Retina.

[10] Frangieh, G. T., W. R. Green, et al. (1981). "A histopathologic study of macular cysts and holes." Retina 1(4): 311-336.

[11] Funata, M., R. T. Wendel, et al. (1992). "Clinicopathologic study of bilateral macular holes treated with pars plana vitrectomy and gas tamponade." Retina 12(4): 289-298.

[12] Gass, J. D. (1988). "Idiopathic senile macular hole. Its early stages and pathogenesis." Arch Ophthalmol 106(5): 629-639.

[13] Gass, J. D. (1995). "Reappraisal of biomicroscopic classification of stages of development of a macular hole." Am J Ophthalmol 119(6): 752-759.

[14] Gentile, R. C., G. Landa, et al. (2010). "Macular hole formation, progression, and surgical repair: case series of serial optical coherence tomography and time lapse morphing video study." BMC Ophthalmol 10: 24.

[15] Haouchine, B., P. Massin, et al. (2004). "Diagnosis of macular pseudoholes and lamellar macular holes by optical coherence tomography." Am J Ophthalmol 138(5): 732-739.

[16] Hayashi, A., T. Yagou, et al. (2011). "Intraoperative changes in idiopathic macular holes by spectral-domain optical coherence tomography." Case Report Ophthalmol 2(2): 149-154.

[17] Ikuno, Y., K. Sayanagi, et al. (2003). "Optical coherence tomographic findings of macular holes and retinal detachment after vitrectomy in highly myopic eyes." Am J Ophthalmol 136(3): 477-481.

[18] Johnson, R. N. and J. D. Gass (1988). "Idiopathic macular holes. Observations, stages of formation, and implications for surgical intervention." Ophthalmology 95(7): 917-924.

[19] Johnson, R. N., H. R. McDonald, et al. (2001). "Traumatic macular hole: observations, pathogenesis, and results of vitrectomy surgery." Ophthalmology 108(5): 853-857.

[20] Jumper, J. M., R. P. Gallemore, et al. (2000). "Features of macular hole closure in the early postoperative period using optical coherence tomography." Retina 20(3): 232-237.

[21] Kang, S. W., K. Ahn, et al. (2003). "Types of macular hole closure and their clinical implications." Br J Ophthalmol 87(8): 1015-1019.

[22] Kelly, N. E. and R. T. Wendel (1991). "Vitreous surgery for idiopathic macular holes. Results of a pilot study." Arch Ophthalmol 109(5): 654-659.

[23] Kobayashi, H., K. Kobayashi, et al. (2002). "Macular hole and myopic refraction." Br J Ophthalmol 86(11): 1269-1273.

[24] Lee, S. H., K. H. Park, et al. (2010). "Secondary macular hole formation after vitrectomy." Retina 30(7): 1072-1077.

[25] Lee, S. W., S. W. Kang, et al. (2011). "Vitreous surgery for impending macular hole." Retina 31(5): 909-914.

[26] Lois, N., J. Burr, et al. (2011). "Internal limiting membrane peeling versus no peeling for idiopathic full thickness macular hole: a pragmatic randomized controlled trial." Invest Ophthalmol Vis Sci 52(3): 1586-1592.

[27] Masuyama, K., K. Yamakiri, et al. (2009). "Posturing time after macular hole surgery modified by optical coherence tomography images: a pilot study." Am J Ophthalmol 147(3): 481-488 e482.

[28] McCannel, C. A., J. L. Ensminger, et al. (2009). "Population-based incidence of macular holes." Ophthalmology 116(7): 1366-1369.

[29] McDonnell, P. J., S. L. Fine, et al. (1982). "Clinical features of idiopathic macular cysts and holes." Am J Ophthalmol 93(6): 777-786.

[30] Menchini, U., G. Virgili, et al. (2003). "Mechanism of spontaneous closure of traumatic macular hole: OCT study of one case." Retina 23(1): 104-106.

[31] Nishimura, A., M. Kimura, et al. (2011). "Efficacy of primary silicone oil tamponade for the treatment of retinal detachment caused by macular hole in high myopia." Am J Ophthalmol 151(1): 148-155.

[32] Oster, S. F., F. Mojana, et al. (2010). "Dynamics of the macular hole-silicone oil tamponade interface with patient positioning as imaged by spectral domain-optical coherence tomography." Retina 30(6): 924-929.

[33] Park, D. W., J. O. Sipperley, et al. (1999). "Macular hole surgery with internal-limiting membrane peeling and intravitreous air." Ophthalmology 106(7): 1392-1397; discussion 1397-1398.

[34] Patel, S. C., R. H. Loo, et al. (2001). "Macular hole surgery in high myopia." Ophthalmology 108(2): 377-380.

[35] Sano, M., M. Inoue, et al. (2011). "Ability to determine postoperative status of macular hole in gas-filled eyes by spectral domain-optical coherence tomography." Clin Experiment Ophthalmol.

[36] Sano, M., Y. Shimoda, et al. (2009). "Restored photoreceptor outer segment and visual recovery after macular hole closure." Am J Ophthalmol 147(2): 313-318 e311.

[37] Shimada, N., K. Ohno-Matsui, et al. (2006). "Natural course of macular retinoschisis in highly myopic eyes without macular hole or retinal detachment." Am J Ophthalmol 142(3): 497-500.

[38] Shimozono, M., A. Oishi, et al. (2011). "Restoration of the photoreceptor outer segment and visual outcomes after macular hole closure: spectral-domain optical coherence tomography analysis." Graefes Arch Clin Exp Ophthalmol.

[39] Sun, C. B., Z. Liu, et al. (2010). "Natural evolution from macular retinoschisis to full thickness macular hole in highly myopic eyes." Eye (Lond) 24(12): 1787-1791.

[40] Takahashi, A., T. Nagaoka, et al. (2010). "Foveal anatomic changes in a progressing stage 1 macular hole documented by spectral-domain optical coherence tomography." Ophthalmology 117(4): 806-810.

[41] Takahashi, A., T. Nagaoka, et al. (2011). "Stage 1-A macular hole: a prospective spectral-domain optical coherence tomography study." Retina 31(1): 127-147.

[42] Takahashi, H. and S. Kishi (1999). "Optical coherence tomography images of spontaneous macular hole closure." Am J Ophthalmol 128(4): 519-520.

[43] Takahashi, H. and S. Kishi (2000). "Tomographic features of a lamellar macular hole formation and a lamellar hole that progressed to a full thickness macular hole." Am J Ophthalmol 130(5): 677-679.

[44] Takahashi, H. and S. Kishi (2000). "Tomographic features of early macular hole closure after vitreous surgery." Am J Ophthalmol 130(2): 192-196.

[45] Takano, M. and S. Kishi (1999). "Foveal retinoschisis and retinal detachment in severely myopic eyes with posterior staphyloma." Am J Ophthalmol 128(4): 472-476.

[46] Tanaka, Y., N. Shimada, et al. (2011). "Natural history of lamellar macular holes in highly myopic eyes." Am J Ophthalmol 152(1): 96-99 e91.

[47] Tornambe, P. E., L. S. Poliner, et al. (1998). "Definition of macular hole surgery end points: elevated/open, flat/open, flat/closed." Retina 18(3): 286-287.

[48] Weichel, E. D. and M. H. Colyer (2009). "Traumatic macular holes secondary to combat ocular trauma." Retina 29(3): 349-354.

[49] Wendel, R. T., A. C. Patel, et al. (1993). "Vitreous surgery for macular holes." Ophthalmology 100(11): 1671-1676.

[50] Wu, T. T. and Y. H. Kung (2011). "Comparison of anatomical and visual outcomes of macular hole surgery in patients with high myopia vs. non-high myopia: a case-control study using optical coherence tomography." Graefes Arch Clin Exp Ophthalmol.

[51] Yamada, H., A. Sakai, et al. (2002). "Spontaneous closure of traumatic macular hole." Am J Ophthalmol 134(3): 340-347.

[52] Yamashita, T., A. Uemara, et al. (2002). "Spontaneous closure of traumatic macular hole." Am J Ophthalmol 133(2): 230-235.

[53] Yeh, P. T., T. C. Chen, et al. (2010). "Formation of idiopathic macular hole-reappraisal." Graefes Arch Clin Exp Ophthalmol 248(6): 793-798.

[54] Yuzawa, M., A. Watanabe, et al. (1994). "Observation of idiopathic full thickness macular holes. Follow-up observation." Arch Ophthalmol 112(8): 1051-1056.

Chapter 4

Optical Coherence Tomography in Neuro-Ophthalmology

Tony Garcia, Ghislain Bonnay, Ayman Tourbah and
Carl Arndt

Additional information is available at the end of the chapter

http://dx.doi.org/10.5772/53510

1. Introduction

In optic nerve disease excluding glaucoma, mainly three ophthalmoscopic presentations of the optic disc can be encountered: an apparently normal optic disc, an atrophic or an edematous optic disc. Many documentation methods in optic neuropathy (ON) have been used: drawings; color, monochromatic and angiographic photographs.

The optical coherence tomography (OCT), based on interferometry analysis, is a major achievement particularly for documentation of quantitative changes in the optic nerve head: it allows a measure of the retinal nerve fiber layer thickness (RNFL). This retinal layer is composed of non myelinated axons (myelination is generally posterior to the cribriform lamina). OCT can quantify a decrease in thickness due to the atrophy by axonal loss or increase in thickness related to edema. This review aims to illustrate the usefulness of this RNFL quantification in the exploration of optic nerve and anterior visual pathway diseases.

2. Materials and methods

An extensive review of the literature on applications of OCT in optic neuropathy was performed. The PubMed search engine was applied to the keywords "optic neuropathy", "optical coherence tomography" and "retinal nerve fiber layer". Studies exploring the various diseases of the optic nerve were classified according to the OCT results obtained at the initial visit. Glaucomatous neuropathy was excluded from this review. Characteristic diseases are illustrated by clinical case reports.

3. Results

The average RNFL thickness is the most common parameter encountered in all publications. It represents the average of all measured thickness values in a predefined annular zone adjacent to the optic disc. In some publications, the macular volume has also been evaluated.

The change over time of the average RNFL thickness could be characterized by two different patterns:

- a normal RNFL thickness at the initial visit, followed by a gradual decrease: progressive RNFL decrease
- an increased RNFL thickness at the initial visit.

4. Progressive decrease of RNFL thickness (evolution towards atrophy)

4.1. Inflammatory diseases: Multiple sclerosis (case reports 1 et 2)

Multiple sclerosis (MS) is the most common cause of optic neuropathy, therefore the evaluation of RNFL thickness in MS was the subject of numerous publications [1,2]

At the initial stage of optic neuritis, RNFL thickness is within normal limits, after 2 months it decreases and stabilizes between 6 and 12 months [3,4] as highlighted in case report 1.

Case report 1:

A 35 year-old man was admitted for subacute left monocular impairment. Left orbital pain increased by ocular movements was reported. Visual acuity was 1.0 on the right eye and 0.4 in the left eye.

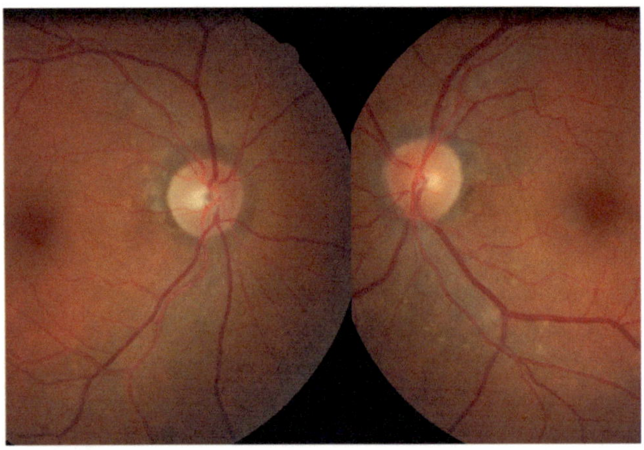

Figure 1. Retinal colour photography (case 1)

http://dx.doi.org/10.5772/53510

Ophthalmoscopy noted normal appearance of the right optic disc and slight left optic disc hyperhemia (figure 1). Acute optic neuritis was suspected. On the OCT, there is a slight RNFL swelling in its nasal superior part, however the mean thickness remains within normal limits (figure 2).

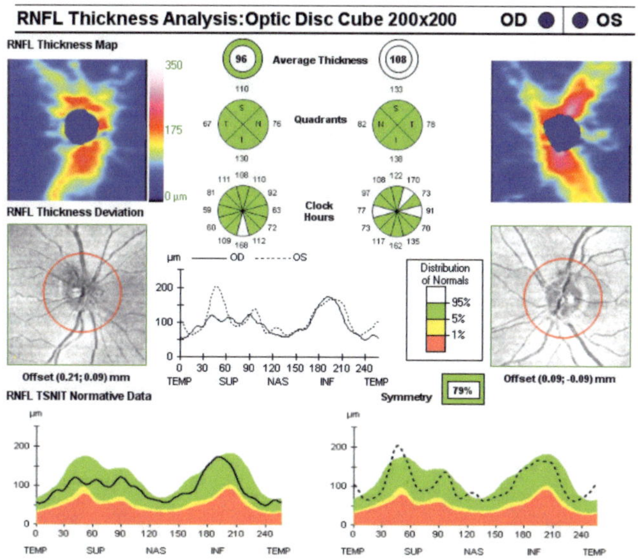

Figure 2. OCT slight RNFL swelling in the left eye (case 1)

The left visual field was abnormal with a nasal inferior defect, the right visual field was normal (figure 3).

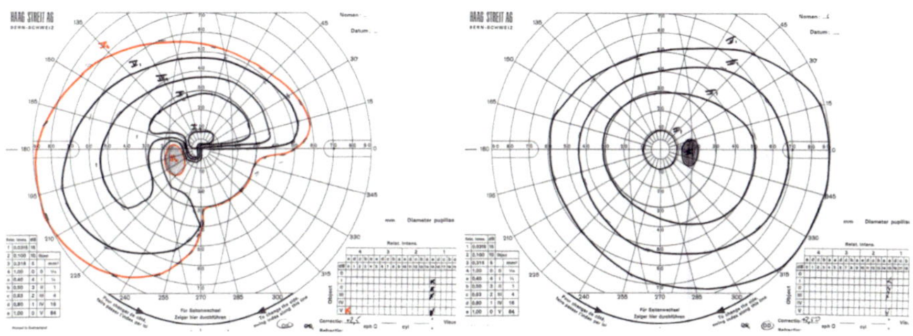

Figure 3. Visual fields (case 1)

After stabilization of the affected eye following an episode of optic neuritis, average RNFL thickness is between 59.75 and 85.00 µm. In the contralateral eye, this parameter is between 82.73 and 99.80 µm (normal range: 102.90 - 111.10 µm) [5]. Thus, axonal loss is often present in both eyes even if symptomatic optic neuritis affects one eye only.

Case report 2

A 54-year-old woman suffered from multiple sclerosis and had already a left demyelinating optic neuritis a few years ago. Flair-weighted axial magnetic resonance image shows periventricular plaques (figure 4).

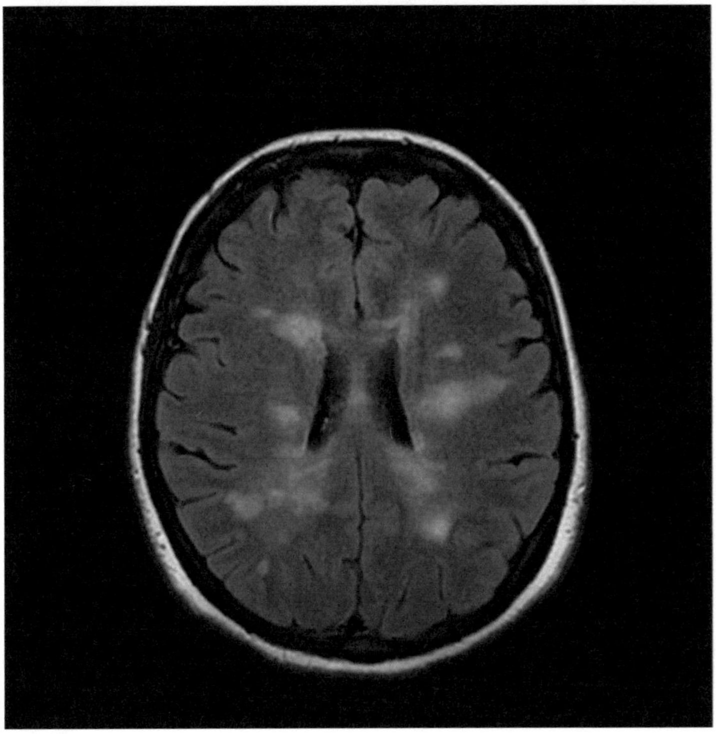

Figure 4. Brain MRI scan (case 2)

Visual acuity was 1.0 in both eyes. Left visual field displayed a small inferior central defect.

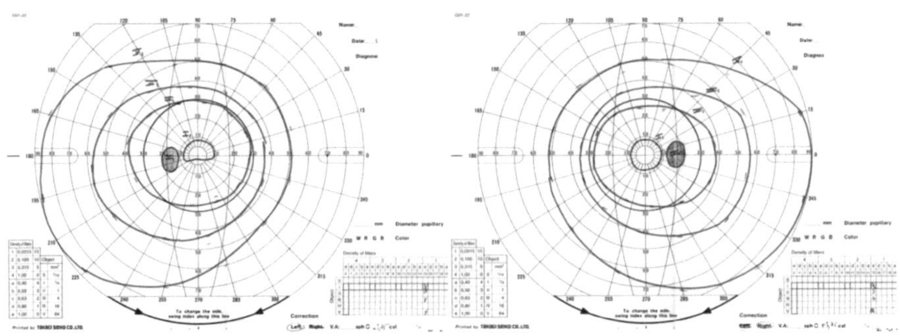

Figure 5. Visual field (case 2)

http://dx.doi.org/10.5772/53510

On ophthalmoscopy, a left temporal disc pallor indicative of previous optic neuritis was noted (figure 6).

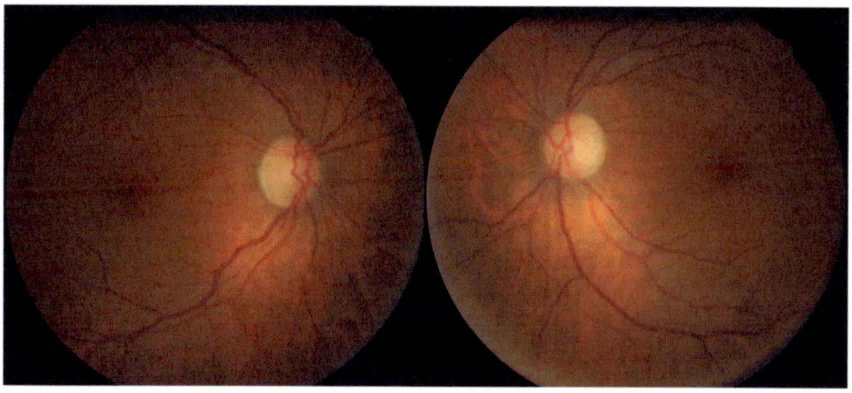

Figure 6. Retinal colour photography: left optic disc pallor (case 2)

OCT could confirm the decrease of the left temporal RNFL (figure 7).

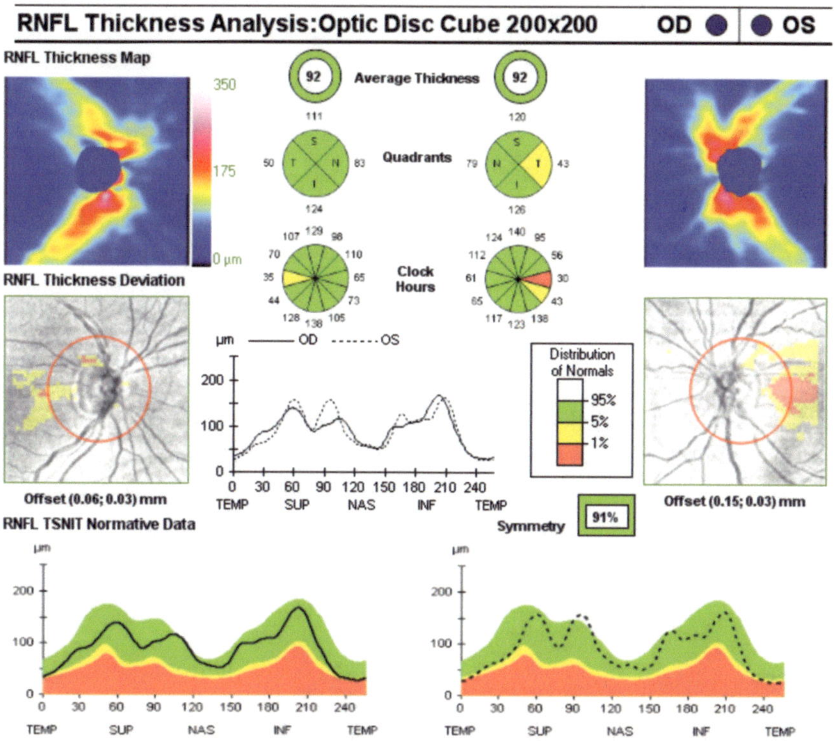

Figure 7. OCT: temporal RNFL thinning (case 2)

However, the importance of RNFL loss depends on the severity of MS in which optic neuritis occurs.

In the eye affected by inaugural optic neuritis, the RNFL thickness stabilizes at 58.10 microns, and at 101.20 microns in the contralateral eye.

If optic neuritis occurs in patients presenting with a relapsing form of MS, RNFL loss is greater in the affected eye, stabilizing at an average thickness of 48.20 μm whereas the contralateral eye remains unaffected, the thickness remains at a high average level of 103.70 μm.

In secondary progressive forms, characterized by a continuous evolution toward a severe neurological disability, axonal loss is even greater in the affected eye of optic neuritis (39.50 μm on average), but also affects the contralateral eye (83.40 μm on average) [6]. This RNFL loss predominates in the temporal quadrant [3] [7], a clinical model demonstrating the coexistence of axonal loss and demyelinating lesions in MS.

Other parameters have been evaluated with OCT in MS, especially a decrease in macular volume which is correlated with axonal loss [8] [9]. The relationship between central and peripheral macular thickness is an indicator of the evolution of the disease [10]. In addition, in MS, RNFL loss is considered to be a fairly accurate indicator of overall axonal loss, both ocular and extraocular. In the early course of the disease, there is a correlation between the decrease in RNFL thickness and neurological disability assessed by the Expanded Disability Status Scale (EDSS) [11] which represents the global axonal loss in MS. There is a relationship between RNFL loss and brain atrophy [12]. Thus RNFL thickness also appears as a reliable marker of disease severity.

Finally, some correlations between OCT parameters and morphological and functional data have been reported.

At the initial stage of optic neuritis: when RNFL thickness is often normal, visual evoked potentials (VEP) (and MRI when it is rapidly accessible) is more efficient to objectify the optic nerve lesions (eliminating a pithiatism when there is a doubt). Thus, at the early stages of MS, OCT is less sensitive than VEP for detecting clinical and subclinical optic neuropathy [13].

At distance of the initial attack of optic neuritis

- there is no correlation between RNFL thickness (a marker of axonal loss) and P100 latency (a marker of demyelination) [14]. In optic neuritis, the increase of cup/disc ratio is inversely proportional to the decrease in visual acuity and the decrease in RNFL thickness [15];
- there is a correlation between RNFL thickness (morphological marker of axonal loss) and visual acuity (a loss of one line of visual acuity corresponds to an average decrease of 5,40 μm in thickness) [16], pattern electroretinogram or pupillary reflex (functional markers of axonal loss) [17, 18].

4.2. Degenerative diseases: Neuromyelitis Optica (NMO) or Devic's disease (case report 3)

In Devic's syndrome, unlike MS, optic neuropathy is severe and is associated with spinal cord lesions without brain damage (figure 10). In OCT, the significant decrease in the thickness of the layer of ganglion fibers reflects an atrophy more severe and diffuse than that observed in MS, mainly in the upper and lower quadrants [19,20]. As in MS, there is a correlation between the retinal nerve fiber layer thickness and the overall neurological disability assessed by the EDSS [21]. OCT can thus provide morphological arguments in the differential diagnosis of Devic's syndrome and MS. In a comparative study, the average thickness was 63.60 μm in Devic's syndrome, whereas it is 88.30 μm in MS (102.00 μm in the group of MS patients in an eye with no history of optic neuropathy) [22]. The average RNFL loss is 15 μm in a patient suffering from MS, whereas it is 39.00 μm in the case of Devic's syndrome [22].

Case 3

A 35-year-old woman had bilateral optic neuritis. Left visual acuity was 1.0. Despite anti-inflammatory treatment, right visual acuity had not recovered and remained very low (0.02).

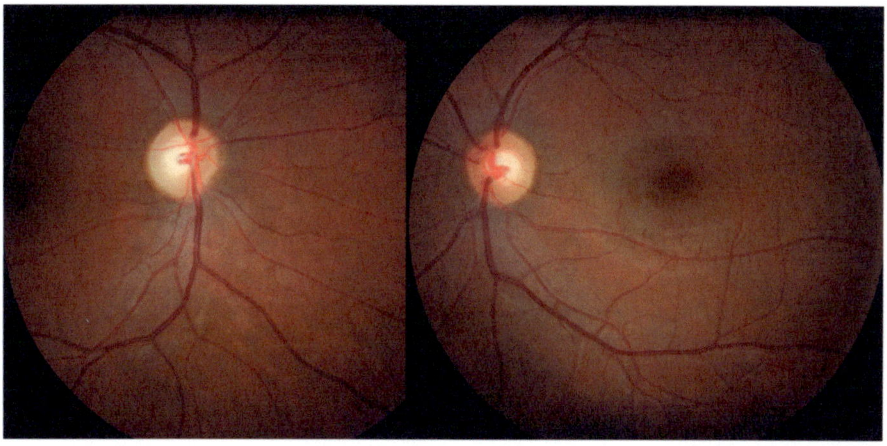

Figure 8. Retinal colour photography (case 3)

Optic atrophy is observed in the right eye, there is an optic disc pallor in the left eye (figure 8)

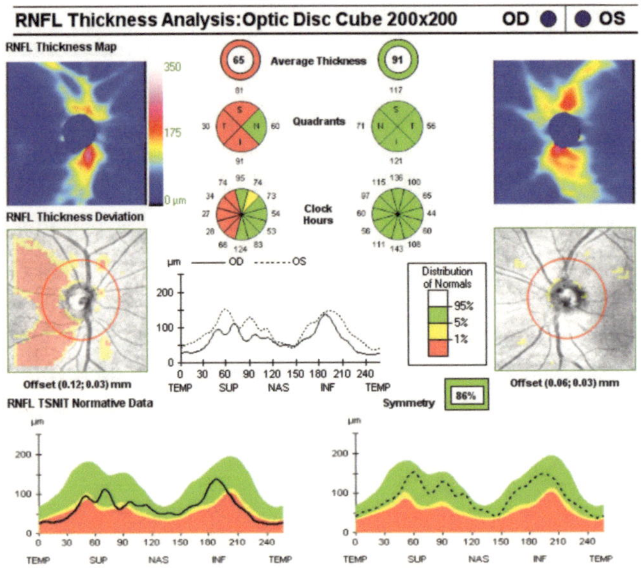

Figure 9. OCT RNFL: loss in the right eye (case 3)

Important decrease of retinal fiber layer was found on the right OCT with an average thickness of 65 µm (figure 9).

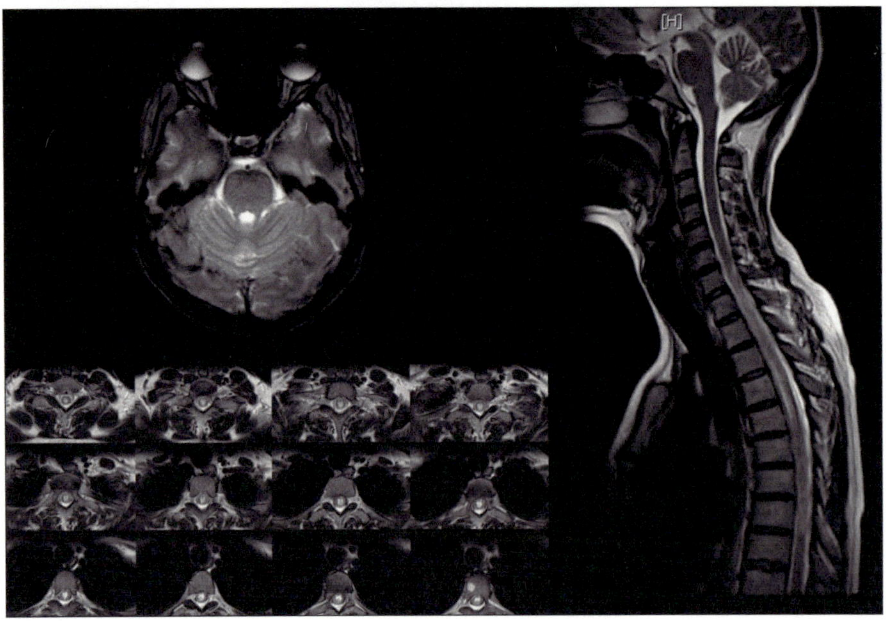

Figure 10. Brain and Medullar MRI scan (case 3)

http://dx.doi.org/10.5772/53510

Transverse myelitis was found on the MRI scan (Figure 10) as part of Devic's disease.

4.3. Compressive disease (case 4)

Compression of visual pathways caused by a pituitary adenoma induces axonal loss responsible for RNFL loss on time domain OCT. The importance of this axonal loss predicts visual acuity changes and visual field recovery after surgery for pituitary adenoma [23]. The postoperative recovery is significantly better if the preoperative thickness is greater than 85.00 µm [24].

Case 4

A 75 year-old man complained of chronic headache. Visual acuity was 0.8 on the right eye and 0.4 in the left one.

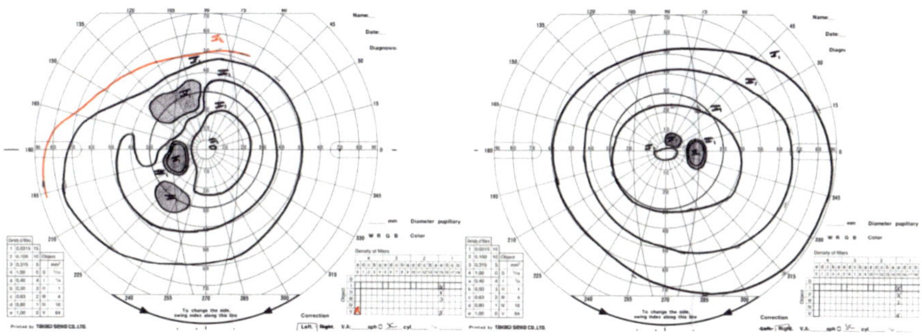

Figure 11. Visual field: temporal asymmetric defect in both eyes (case 4)

Visual fields showed temporal defects in particular in the left field (Figure 11).

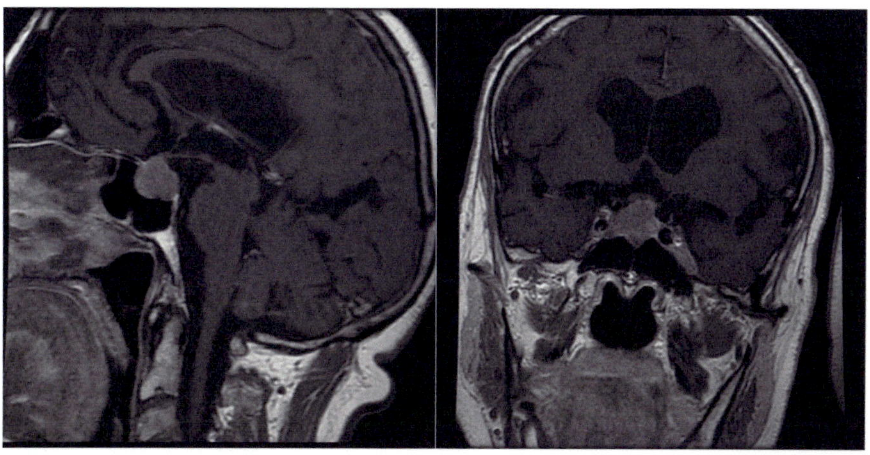

Figure 12. Brain MRI scan (case 4)

Magnetic resonance imaging discovered a large pituitary tumor with chiasm compression (figure 12).

Preoperative average RNFL thickness attests of significant axonal loss in the temporal area.

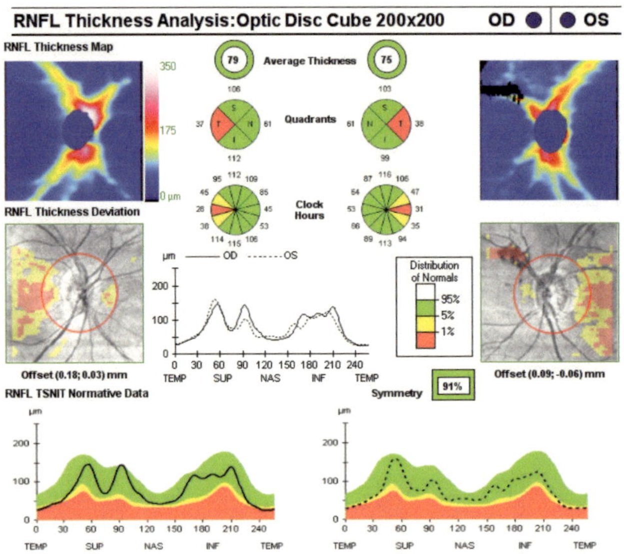

Figure 13. OCT: temporal RNFL thinning (case 4)

4.4. Hereditary disease

4.4.1. Dominant Optic Atrophy (DOA) or Kjer's disease (Case 5)

In dominant optic atrophy (DOA), there is bilateral symmetric optic nerve pallor (Case 5) related to retinal ganglion cell death. The decrease in the RNFL thickness in OCT is dominant in the temporal part [25].

Case 5

A seven year old girl is referred for poor visual acuity (RE 20/40, LE 20/50) associated with bilateral optic disc atrophy (Figure 14).

http://dx.doi.org/10.5772/53510

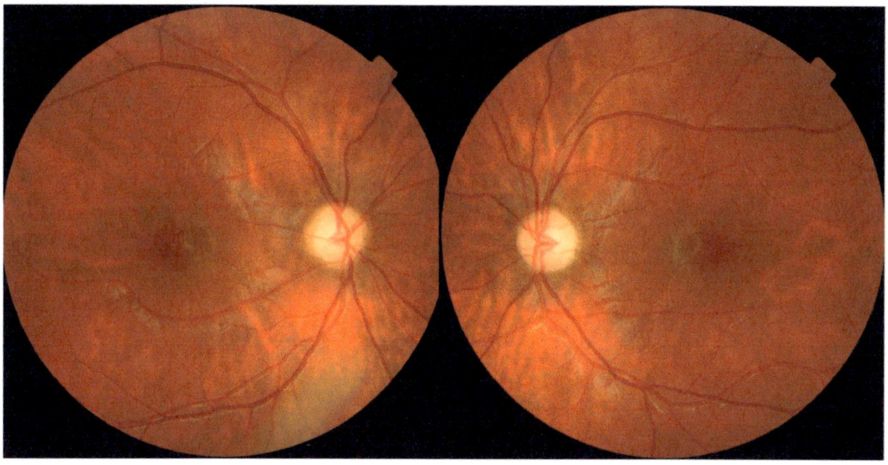

Figure 14. Retinal colour photography (case 5): bilateral optic atrophy

On color vision testing there is a blue-yellow confusion axis (Figure 15).

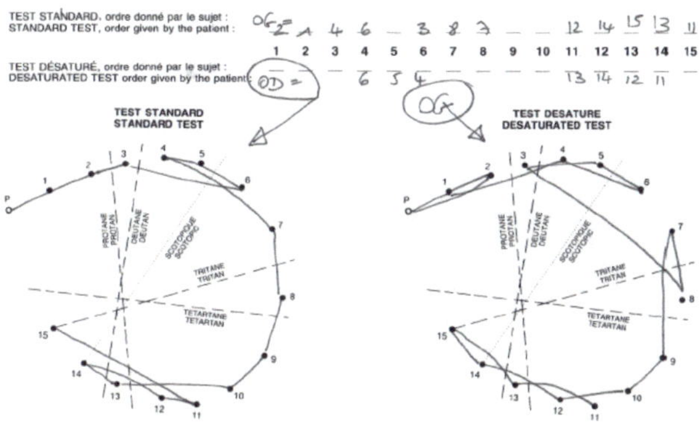

Figure 15. Farnsworth 15HUE (case 5): yellow blue defect

On the time domain OCT, a major bilateral RNFL loss is noted (Figure 16).

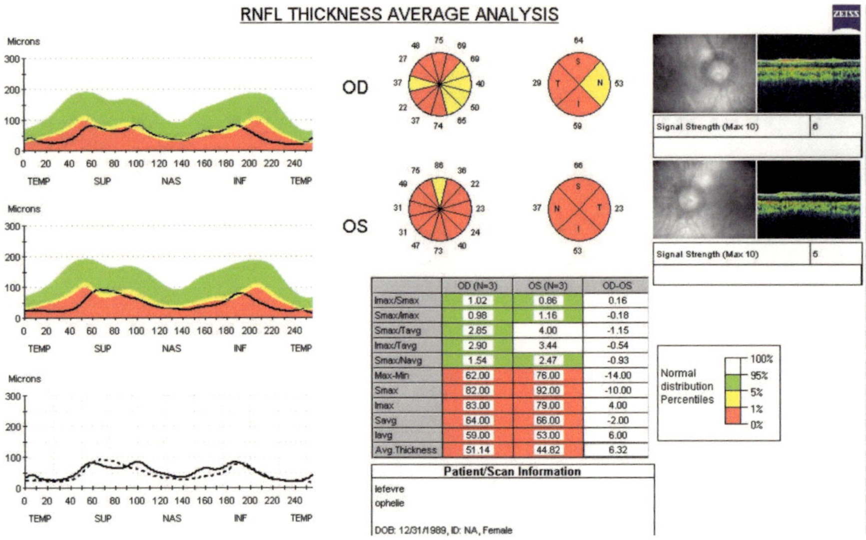

Figure 16. OCT: RNFL loss in both eyes (case 5)

There is no compressive process on the brain MRI which only displays atrophic optic nerves (figure 17).

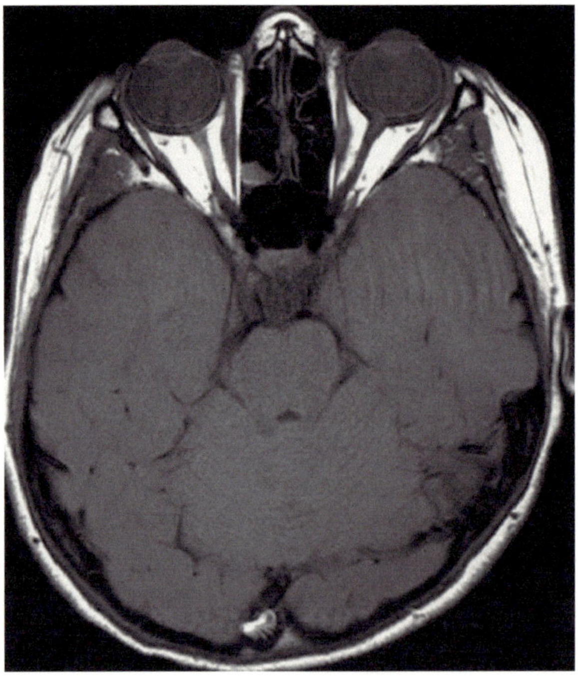

Figure 17. Brain MRI scan (case 5): bilateral thinning of the optic nerves

http://dx.doi.org/10.5772/53510

A dominant pattern was found upon family enquiry (Figure 18).

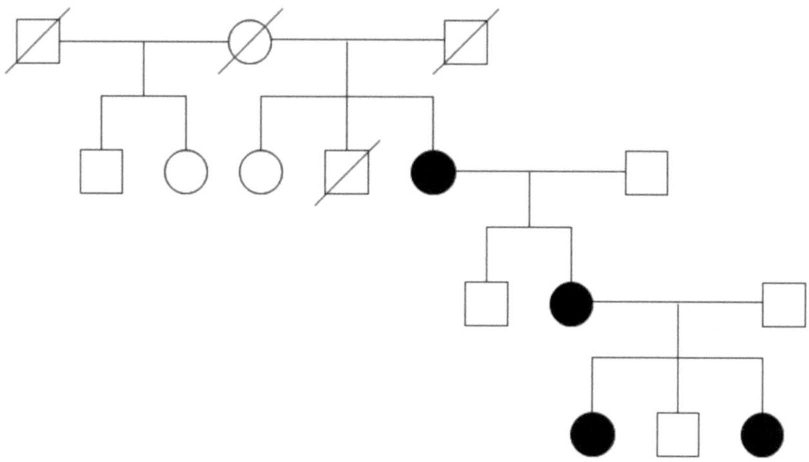

Figure 18. Family enquiry (case 5)

4.4.2. Other hereditary optic neuropathies

In the authors' clinical experience, OCT is also useful in the morphological evaluation of optic neuropathies encountered in other hereditary diseases such as recessive optic neuropathy and Wolfram's disease. However no reports on this subject could be found.

4.5. Toxic optic neuropathy

OCT can be useful for the follow-up of visual loss in patients with toxic optic neuropathy due to smoking, alcohol consumption or treatment for tuberculosis. In the early stages of toxic optic neuropathy, RNFL edema may be detected in some patients before permanent visual loss occurs. RNFL decrease consecutive to the withdrawal of the toxic agent can be monitored with OCT.

Case 6

A 48-year-old woman complained of progressive and painless visual loss. She had alcohol and tobacco addiction. She was deficient in B vitamins. Visual acuity was 0.3 in the right eye and 0.4 in the left eye. Color fundus photos showed pale optic discs without hemorrhage. Miliary drusens were also observed on macular areas (Figure 19).

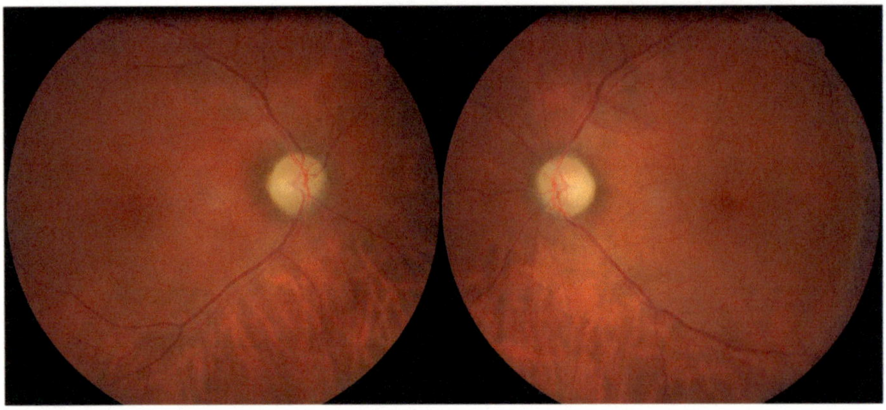

Figure 19. Retinal colour photography (case 6): bilateral optic atrophy

Centrocaecal scotomas were visible in both visual fields (Figure 20)

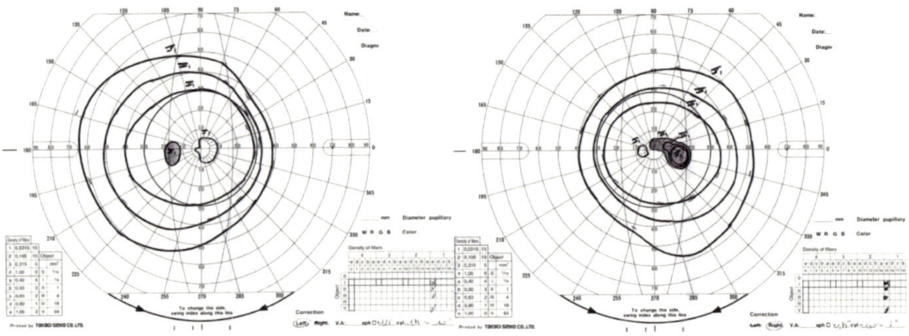

Figure 20. Visual fields (case 6)

OCT confirmed optic nerve atrophy demonstrating a global RNFL loss.

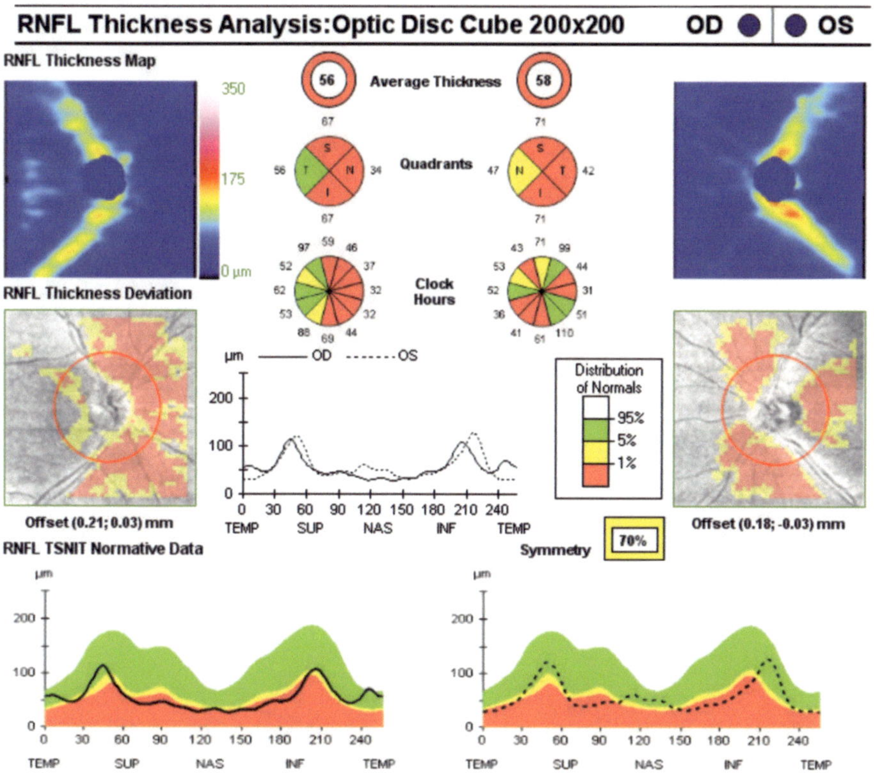

Figure 21. OCT RNFL: loss in both eyes (case 6)

5. Gradual RNFL reduction following initial increase of RNFL thickness

In optic disc swelling, an increase in the RNFL thickness can be quantified by OCT.

Depending on the underlying disease, the condition will either resolve with normalization or shift to optic atrophy with axonal loss. This evolution can be monitored with OCT.

5.1. Papilledema (case 7)

Optic disc swelling due to idiopathic intracranial hypertension is referred to as papilledema [26]. It may be responsible for the deterioration of visual function and progression to optic atrophy. Visual field and VEP are prognostic indicators for visual outcome [27]. This is not the case for RNFL thickness changes which only enable to monitor the progression of the disease.

Case 7

A 28-year-old woman suffered from headache and vomiting. On ophthalmologic examination, visual acuity was 0.9 on the right eye and 1.0 on the left eye without oculomotor paralysis. This condition was due to intracranial hypertension. A bilateral papilloedema, venous engorgement, white exudates and superficial retinal folds was found (Figure 22).

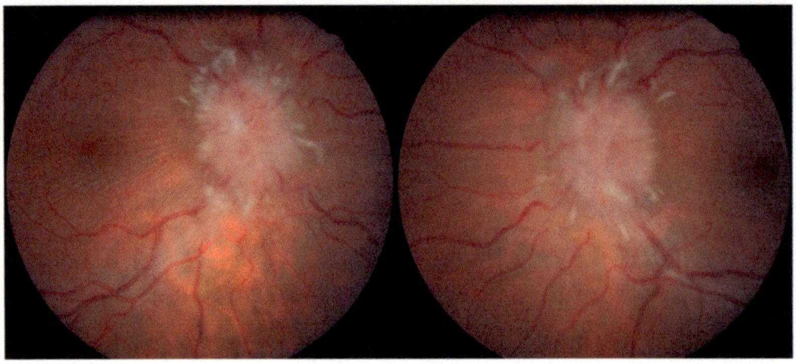

Figure 22. Retinal colour photography (case 7): bilateral optic nerve head swelling

Blind spots were enlarged on visual fields (figure 23).

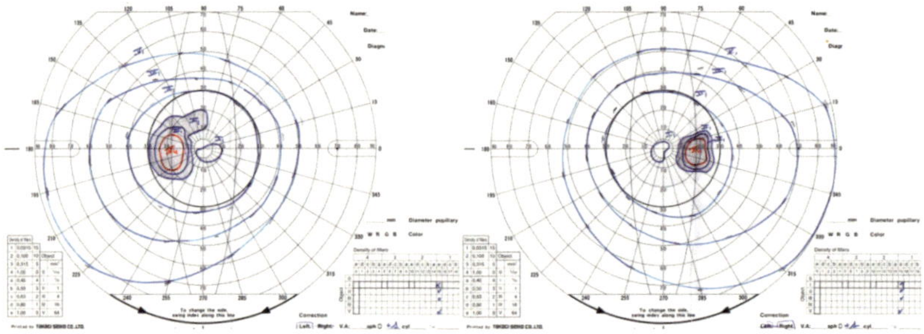

Figure 23. Visual fields (case 7)

After spinal puncture and acetazolamide medication, she recovered normal visual acuity. OCT follow-up enabled to monitor the improvement with treatment (Figure 24).

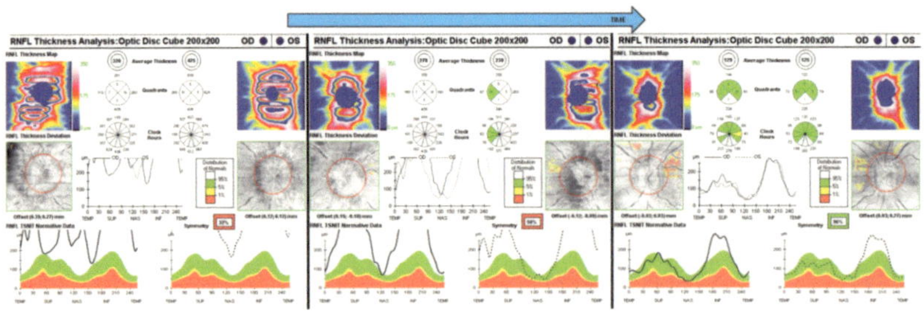

Figure 24. OCT RNFL follow-up (case 7)

5.2. Anterior Ischemic Optic Neuropathy (AION)

At the initial stage of an anterior ischemic optic neuropathy, there is most often a progressive optic disc swelling. Then, axonal loss is responsible for a gradual reduction of RNFL leading to a variable stage of optic atrophy stabilizing at six months of onset [28].

5.3. Leber's Hereditary Optic Neuropathy (LHON) (case 8)

At the acute phase, Leber's hereditary optic neuropathy associates peripapillary telangiectasia, tortuosity of retinal vessels and a peripapillary RNFL swelling with apparent optic disc swelling (figure 25-27). Within a few months (generally less than six months), diffuse optic atrophy occurs without excavation [29,30].

Case 8

An 11-year-old girl with no family history of Leber's disease suddenly presented with severe painless central vision loss in the right eye. Dilated capillaries in the retina adjacent to the optic nerve head were found in both eyes. Two months after onset, visual acuity in the left eye also decreased.

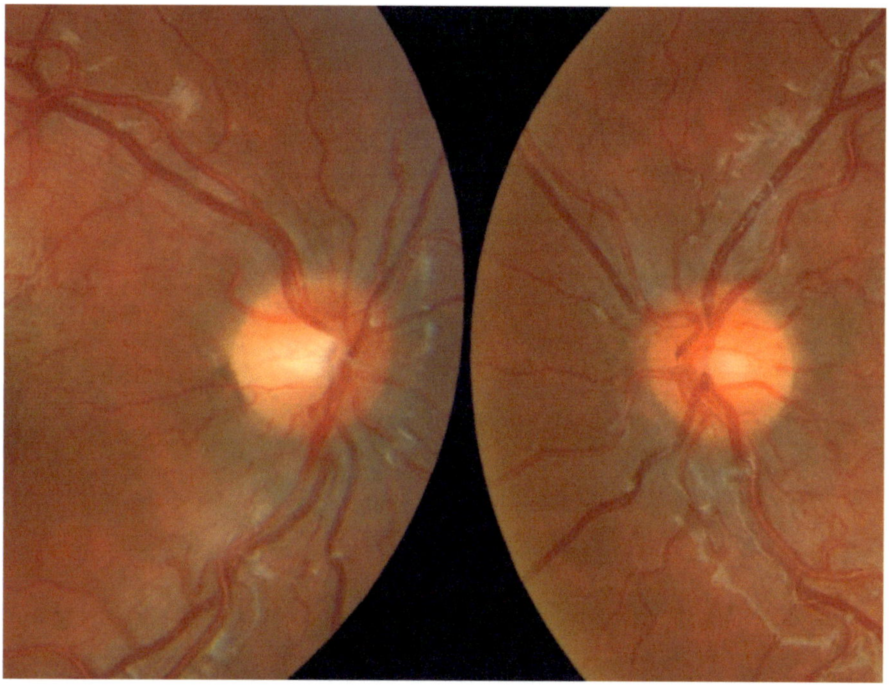

Figure 25. Retinal colour photography (case 8)

Average RNFL thickness was increased in both eyes on the initial examination and it then slowly decreased as optic atrophy developed.

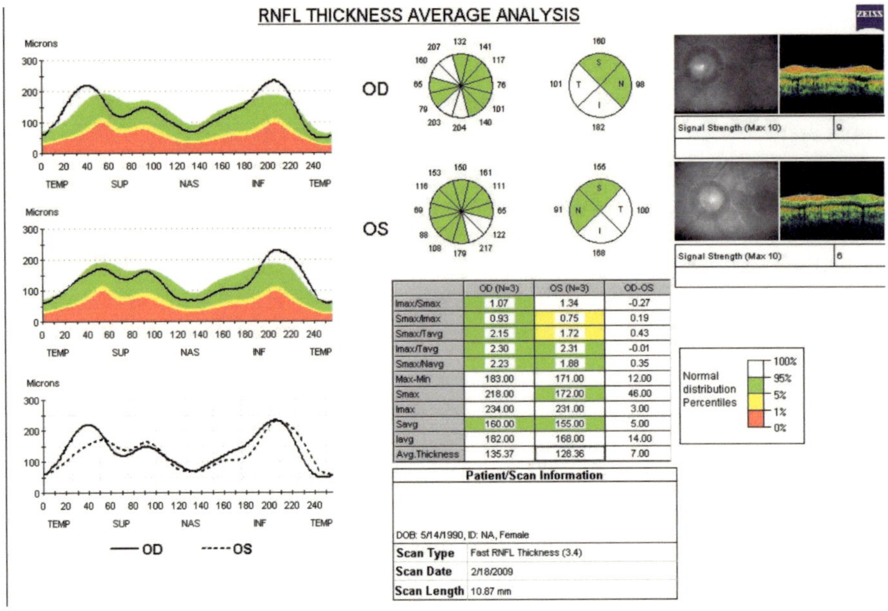

	OD (N=3)	OS (N=3)	OD-OS
Imax/Smax	1.07	1.34	-0.27
Smax/Imax	0.93	0.75	0.19
Smax/Tavg	2.15	1.72	0.43
Imax/Tavg	2.30	2.31	-0.01
Smax/Navg	2.23	1.88	0.35
Max-Min	183.00	171.00	12.00
Smax	218.00	172.00	46.00
Imax	234.00	231.00	3.00
Savg	160.00	155.00	5.00
Iavg	182.00	168.00	14.00
Avg.Thickness	135.37	128.36	7.00

Patient/Scan Information	
DOB: 5/14/1990, ID: NA, Female	
Scan Type	Fast RNFL Thickness (3.4)
Scan Date	2/18/2009
Scan Length	10.87 mm

Figure 26. Initial OCT RNFL (case 8)

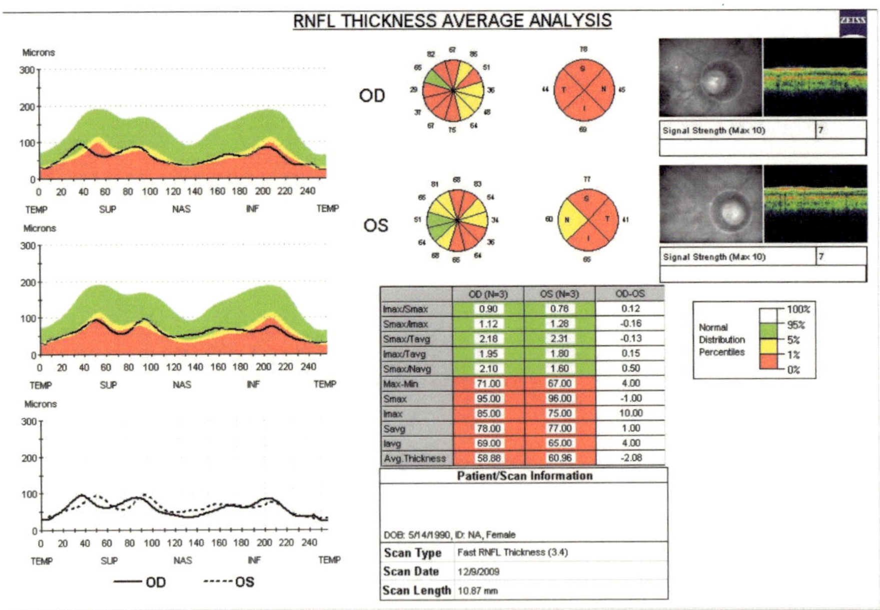

	OD (N=3)	OS (N=3)	OD-OS
Imax/Smax	0.90	0.78	0.12
Smax/Imax	1.12	1.28	-0.16
Smax/Tavg	2.18	2.31	-0.13
Imax/Tavg	1.95	1.80	0.15
Smax/Navg	2.10	1.60	0.50
Max-Min	71.00	67.00	4.00
Smax	95.00	96.00	-1.00
Imax	85.00	75.00	10.00
Savg	78.00	77.00	1.00
Iavg	69.00	65.00	4.00
Avg.Thickness	58.88	60.96	-2.08

Patient/Scan Information	
DOB: 5/14/1990, ID: NA, Female	
Scan Type	Fast RNFL Thickness (3.4)
Scan Date	12/9/2009
Scan Length	10.87 mm

Figure 27. End stage OCT RNFL (case 8)

5.4. Secondary intracranial hypertension

Many different diseases can be responsible for increased intracranial pressure such as infectious meningitis (case 9). As in other diseases with initial optic disc swelling, OCT enables to monitor RNFL thickness reduction after causal treatment.

Case 9

A 47-year-old man was admitted for visual field disorders with papulosquamous eruption of the palms and soles within two weeks following a previous asymptomatic general skin eruption. Visual acuity was 0.8 in both eyes. Bilateral optic nerve head swelling was observed (figure 28).

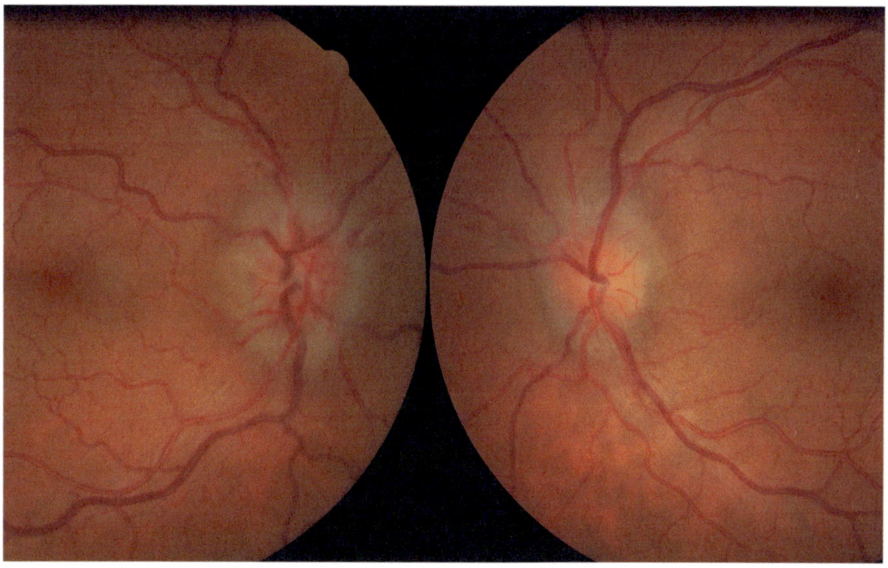

Figure 28. Retinal colour photography (case 9): Optic nerve head swelling

Goldmann visual fields displayed inferior altitudinal field defects (Figure 29).

Serological tests on blood and cerebrospinal fluid confirmed a syphilitic infection. After initial intravenous penicillin G, the patient was discharged with ceftriaxone injections (1 g/day) for three weeks. On the OCT scans, the decrease of optic nerve head swelling was replaced with superior optic atrophy (figure 30).

6. Limitations

Although OCT provides very useful quantitative information on RNFL thickness, there are several limitation inherent to the device which should be highlighted.

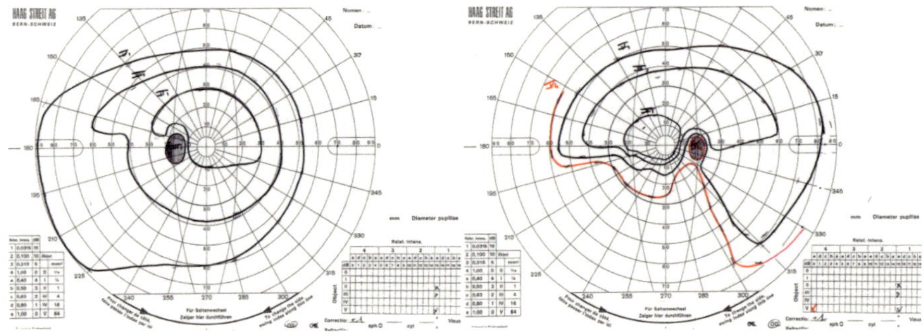

Figure 29. Visual fields (case 9)

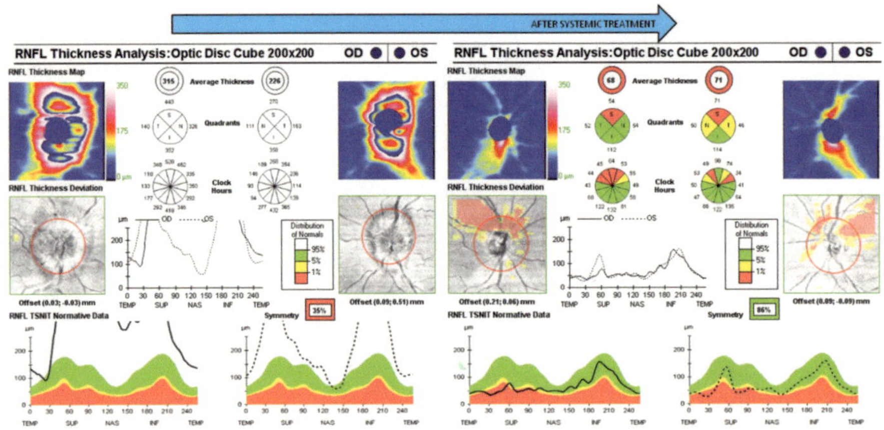

Figure 30. OCT RNFL follow-up (case 9)

6.1. Age

In the OCT database, normal values apply only to patients over 18 years. Evaluation of RNFL thickness is based on the assumption that there are no significant changes in normals from birth to the age of 18.

6.2. Morphological variations

RNFL thickness evaluation by OCT is not a reliable method in case of major morphologic changes of the optic nerve head such peripapillary atrophy in high myopia, staphyloma or optic pits.

6.3. Refractive media disorders

Ultra-red light has to pass through the transparent media of the eye to reach the retina. In case of corneal dystrophy, cataract, vitreous opacity, there is a signal decrease and RNFL thickness measurements become less reliable.

http://dx.doi.org/10.5772/53510

7. Discussion

As in macular disease, OCT has become a precious tool that contributes to improve management of optic nerve disease. This review illustrates the many indications in neuro-ophthalmology, although there are limitations to its use. OCT measures RNFL thickness to assess axonal loss [31]. Axonal loss may be masked in cases with optic nerve head swelling due to the inhibition of orthograde axoplasmic transport at the initial stage of the disease.

Despite the high utility of OCT in neuro-ophthalmology, exclusive RNFL thickness analysis is not sufficient for assessing optic nerve disease. OCT results should always be interpreted in the light of clinical ophthalmoloscopy and visual function (visual acuity, perimetry, visual evoked potentials).

8. Declaration of interest

The authors hereby declare that they have no conflict of interest related to this article.

Author details

Tony Garcia[1], Ghislain Bonnay[2], Ayman Tourbah[3] and Carl Arndt[1]

1 Ophtalmologie, Hôpital Robert Debré, Reims University Hospital, Reims, France

2 Service d'Ophtalmologie, Troyes General Hospital, Troyes, France

3 Service de Neurologie, Hôpital Maison Blanche, Reims University Hospital, Reims, France

References

[1] Garcia-martin, E, Pueyo, V, Martin, J, & Fernandez, F. J. Progressive changes in the retinal nerve fiber layer in patients with multiple sclerosis. Eur J Ophthalmol (2010). , 20, 167-173.

[2] Beddiaf, A, & De Sèze, J. Névrite optique dans la sclérose en plaques : données diagnostiques et pronostiques. Rev Neurol (2009). SS147, 145.

[3] Costello, F, Hodge, W, Pan, Y. I, Eggenberger, E, Coupland, S, & Kardon, R. H. Tracking retinal nerve fiber layer loss after optic neuritis: a prospective study using optical coherence tomography. Mult Scler (2008). , 14, 893-905.

[4] Costello, F, Coupland, S, Hodge, W, Lorello, G. R, Koroluk, J, Pan, Y. I, et al. Quantifying axonal loss after optic neuritis with optical coherence tomography. Ann Neurol (2006). , 59, 963-969.

[5] Kallenbach, K, & Frederiksen, J. Optical coherence tomography in optic neuritis and multiple sclerosis: a review. Eur J Neurol (2007). , 14, 841-849.

[6] Costello, F, Hodge, W, Pan, Y. I, Freedman, M, & Demeulemeester, C. Differences in retinal nerve fiber layer atrophy between multiple sclerosis subtypes. J Neurol Sci (2009). , 281, 74-79.

[7] Pro, M. J, Pons, M. E, Liebmann, J. M, Ritch, R, Zafar, S, Lefton, D, et al. Imaging of the optic disc and retinal nerve fiber layer in acute optic neuritis. J Neurol Sci (2006). , 250, 114-119.

[8] Burkholder, B. M, Osborne, B, Loguidice, M. J, Bisker, E, Frohman, T. C, Conger, A, et al. Macular volume determined by optical coherence tomography as a measure of neuronal loss in multiple sclerosis. Arch Neurol (2009). , 66, 1366-1372.

[9] Pulicken, M, Gordon-lipkin, E, Balcer, L. J, Frohman, E, Cutter, G, & Calabresi, P. A. Optical coherence tomography and disease subtype in multiple sclerosis. Neurology (2007). , 69, 2085-2092.

[10] Gugleta, K, Mehling, M, Kochkorov, A, Grieshaber, M, Katamay, R, Flammer, J, et al. Pattern of macular thickness changes measured by ocular coherence tomography in patients with multiple sclerosis. Klin Monatsbl Augenheilkd (2008). , 225, 408-412.

[11] Outteryck, O, Zephir, H, Defoort, S, Bouyon, M, Debruyne, P, Bouacha, I, et al. Optical coherence tomography in clinically isolated syndrome: no evidence of subclinical retinal axonal loss. Arch Neurol (2009). , 66, 1373-1377.

[12] Siger, M, Dziegielewski, K, Jasek, L, Bieniek, M, Nicpan, A, Nawrocki, J, et al. Optical coherence tomography in multiple sclerosis: thickness of the retinal nerve fiber layer as a potential measure of axonal loss and brain atrophy. J Neurol (2008). , 255, 1555-1560.

[13] Naismith, R. T, Tutlam, N. T, Xu, J, Shepherd, J. B, Klawiter, E. C, Song, S. K, et al. Optical coherence tomography is less sensitive than visual evoked potentials in optic neuritis. Neurology (2009). , 73, 46-52.

[14] Gundogan, F. C, Demirkaya, S, & Sobaci, G. Is optical coherence tomography really a new biomarker candidate in multiple sclerosis? A structural and functional evaluation. Invest Ophthalmol Vis Sci (2007). , 48, 5773-5781.

[15] Rebolleda, G, Noval, S, Contreras, I, Arnalich-montiel, F, García-perez, J. L, & Muñoz-negrete, F. J. Optic disc cupping after optic neuritis evaluated with optic coherence tomography. Eye (2009). , 23, 890-894.

[16] Noval, S, Contreras, I, Rebolleda, G, & Muñoz-negrete, F. J. Optical coherence tomography versus automated perimetry for follow-up of optic neuritis. Acta Ophthalmol Scand (2006). , 84, 790-794.

[17] Parisi, V, Manni, G, Spadaro, M, Colacino, G, Restuccia, R, Marchi, S, et al. Correlation between morphological and functional retinal impairment in multiple sclerosis patients. Invest Ophthalmol Vis Sci (1999). , 40, 2520-2527.

[18] Salter, A. R, Conger, A, Frohman, T. C, Zivadinov, R, Eggenberger, E, Calabresi, P, et al. Retinal architecture predicts pupillary reflex metrics in MS. Mult Scler (2009). , 15, 479-486.

[19] Green, A. J, & Cree, B. A. Distinctive retinal nerve fibre layer and vascular changes in neuromyelitis optica following optic neuritis. J Neurol Neurosurg Psychiatry (2009). , 80, 1002-1005.

[20] Naismith, R. T, Tutlam, N. T, Xu, J, Klawiter, E. C, Shepherd, J, Trinkaus, K, et al. Optical coherence tomography differs in neuromyelitis optica compared with multiple sclerosis. Neurology (2009). , 72, 1077-1082.

[21] De Seze, J, Blanc, F, Jeanjean, L, Zéphir, H, Labauge, P, Bouyon, M, et al. Optical coherence tomography in neuromyelitis optica. Arch Neurol (2008). , 65, 920-923.

[22] Ratchford, J. N, Quigg, M. E, Conger, A, Frohman, T, Frohman, E, Balcer, L. J, et al. Optical coherence tomography helps differentiate neuromyelitis optica and MS optic neuropathies. Neurology (2009). , 73, 302-308.

[23] Savino, P. J. Evaluation of the retinal nerve fiber layer: descriptive or predictive? J Neuroophthalmol (2009). , 29, 245-249.

[24] Danesh-meyer, H. V, Papchenko, T, Savino, P. J, Law, A, Evans, J, & Gamble, G. D. In vivo retinal nerve fiber layer thickness measured by optical coherence tomography predicts visual recovery after surgery for parachiasmal tumors. Invest Ophthalmol Vis Sci (2008). , 49, 1879-1885.

[25] Hamel, C, & Lenaers, G. Neuropathies optiques héréditaires. EMC (Elsevier Masson SAS, Paris), Ophtalmologie, 21-480-E-30, (2007).

[26] Walsh and Hoyt's Clinical Neuro-Ophtalmology PhiladelphiaPA, USA: Lippincott Williams & Wilkins ((1998). , 487-548.

[27] Biousse, V, & Newman, N. J. Management of optic nerve disorders: part II. Idiopathic intracranial hypertension. Drugs Today (1997). , 33, 19-24.

[28] Contreras, I, Noval, S, Rebolleda, G, & Muñoz-negrete, F. J. Follow-up of nonarteritic anterior ischemic optic neuropathy with optical coherence tomography. Ophthalmology (2007). , 114, 2338-2344.

[29] Votruba, M. Inherited optic neuropathies. Pediatric Ophtalmology, Neuro-Ophtalmology, Genetics Berlin: Ed. Springer ((2008). , 51-67.

[30] Subei, A. M, & Eggenberger, E. R. Optical coherence tomography: another useful tool in a neuro-ophthalmologist's armamentarium. Curr Opin Ophthalmol (2009). , 20, 462-466.

[31] Pula, J. H, & Reder, A. T. Multiple sclerosis. Part I: neuro-ophthalmic manifestations. Curr Opin Ophthalmol (2009). , 20, 467-475.

Section 2

Atherosclerosis

Chapter 5

Visualization of Plaque Neovascularization by OCT

Hironori Kitabata and Takashi Akasaka

Additional information is available at the end of the chapter

http://dx.doi.org/10.5772/53051

1. Introduction

Although the introduction of drug-eluting-stents (DES) has dramatically reduced restenosis and the need for repeat revascularization compared with bare-metal stents (BMS), percutaneous coronary intervention (PCI) does not always prevent cardiac events, including acute coronary syndrome (ACS) [1]. Therefore, for all cardiologists, the detection of vulnerable plaques before they rupture is one of ultimate goals to predict and prevent ACS. Vulnerable plaques are characterized as thin fibrous cap (<65 μm), large lipid core, and macrophage infiltration within the cap. Furthermore, plaque neovascularization has been identified recently as a common feature of plaque vulnerability. Increased neovascularization in atherosclerotic plaques plays an important role in plaque progression, plaque instability, and rupture of plaque [2-5]. Until recently, however, in vivo studies assessing neovascularization in atherosclerotic plaques have been difficult because of the lack of sufficient resolution that reliably identifies this feature of vulnerable plaque. The first-generation catheter-based Time-domain optical coherence tomography (TD-OCT) system (M2 and M3 OCT system; LightLab Imaging, Westford, MA, USA), which offers superior resolution of 10-15 μm, has emerged as an intracoronary imaging modality, rendering the detailed micro-structure information of coronary plaques [6-8]. With its excellent resolution, OCT may provide an opportunity to directly detect plaque neovascularization in vivo. This chapter reviews the evidence of plaque neovascularization accumulated so far on OCT and discuss the future perspectives and limitations.

2. Neovascularization in atherosclerosis

Nourishment of normal blood vessels is accomplished by oxygen diffusion from the vessel lumen or from adventitial vasa vasorum [9]. As atherosclerosis progresses, the intima thickens, and oxygen diffusion is impaired. As a result, vasa vasorum proliferates in the inner layers of the vessel wall, and becomes major source of nutrients. Vasa vasorum neovascularization in early atherosclerosis is associated with inflammatory cell infiltration and lipid deposition, leading to plaque progression [10]. Furthermore, intraplaque hemorrhage from microvessels contributes to expansion of the necrotic core through the accumulation of free cholesterol from erythrocyte membranes. Several human pathologic studies have demonstrated that plaque neovascularization is pronounced among patients with unstable coronary syndromes and that its presence may be a marker of plaque instability and plaque rupture [4, 5, 11]. Therefore, investigations of imaging methods with the ability to visualize neovascularization would appear worthwhile.

3. Potential imaging modalities of neovascularization

Several imaging modalities such as micro-computed tomography (CT), magnetic resonance imaging (MRI), and ultrasound have emerged as potential techniques for imaging neovessels in atherosclerotic plaques. Micro-CT provides high-resolution images of coronary vasa vasorum neovascularization and insight into their structure and function in animal models [12, 13]. Winter et al have reported that molecular MRI with $\alpha v\beta 3$-targeted, paramagnetic nanoparticles can detect plaque neovessels in atherosclerotic rabbit model [14]. In addition, more recently, Sirol et al have demonstrated how gadofluorine M-enhanced MRI can accurately identify plaque neovascularization in an animal model of atherosclerosis with good histological correlation [15]. Thus, even though the results from these techniques are promising, further studies are needed for clinical application in humans. Intravascular ultrasound (IVUS) has the potential to detect flow within the plaque and subsequently evaluate functional neovessels. The development of IVUS-based imaging has recently demonstrated the preliminary data imaging neovascularization in coronary plaques in vivo after intravascular injection of microbubbles [16,17], but further investigations will be required to show the feasibility of this method for routine clinical use.

4. Plaque neovascularization by OCT

OCT has been proposed as a high-resolution imaging modality that can identify micro-structures in atherosclerotic plaques [8, 18, 19]. The superb high-resolution of OCT may offer an opportunity of studying the spatial distribution of plaque neovascularization in vivo (Figure 1) [20]. In fact, it has been shown that OCT is able to visualize neovascularization of atherosclerotic plaques [21-24]. In addition, Vorpahl et al demonstrated that small black holes in atheromatous plaques observed by OCT were in good agreement with the pathohistological evidence of intra-plaque neoangiogenesis formation in an autopsy case [25]. We recently assessed the relationship between intra-plaque microchannel structures identified by OCT, probably representing neovascularization, and plaque vulnerability in patients with coronary artery disease [21]. In this study, microchannel was defined as a no-signal tubuloluminal structure that was present on at least 3 consecutive OCT cross-sections in pull-back images. As a result, microchannels were seen in 38% of culprit plaques, and plaques with microchannels displayed the characteristics of vulnerability such as positive remodeling and thin fibrous caps compared with plaques without these structures. Of note, the presence of increased microchannel counts was correlated with a greater frequency of thin-capped fibroatheroma (TCFA) (Figure 2). More recently, in larger study population (356 plaques in 117 patients), Tian et al investigated the clinical significance of intra-plaque neovascularization in culprit lesions and no-culprit lesions of unstable angina pectoris (UAP) and in lesions of stable angina pectoris (SAP) using OCT [22]. Intra-plaque neovascularization was found in 35% of UAP culprit lesions, in 34% of UAP non-culprit lesions, and in 28% of SAP lesions, with no significant difference. Among UAP culprit lesions, plaques with neovessel had thinner fibrous cap thickness (56±20 μm vs. 75±30 μm, p<0.001) and significantly higher incidence of TCFA (81% vs. 47%, p=0.002) compared with those without neovessel. In addition, plaque burden was significantly bigger in UAP culprit lesions with neovascularization (79.8±7.9% vs. 72.8±10.7%, p=0.024). In terms of the non-culprit lesions of UAP patients and lesions of SAP patients, however, no significant difference in plaque characteristics was observed, regardless of the presence or absence of neovascularization. Interestingly, Kato et al reported that although the overall prevalence of microchannel in non-culprit lesions was not significantly different between ACS and non-ACS patients (64.7% versus 55.2%, respectively, P=0.647), the closest distance from the lumen to microchannel was shorter in ACS subjects than in non-ACS (104.6±67.0 μm versus 198.3±133.0 μm, p=0.027) [23]. The authors speculated that because neovascular networks expand from the adventitia into the intima as disease progresses [26], plaques with neovascularization located closer to the lumen might represent an advanced stage of atherosclerosis. Furthermore, Uemura et al revealed that microchannel structure in non-culprit plaques (defined as percent diameter stenosis of < 50%) identified by OCT is a predictor of subsequent plaque progression in patients with coronary artery disease [24].

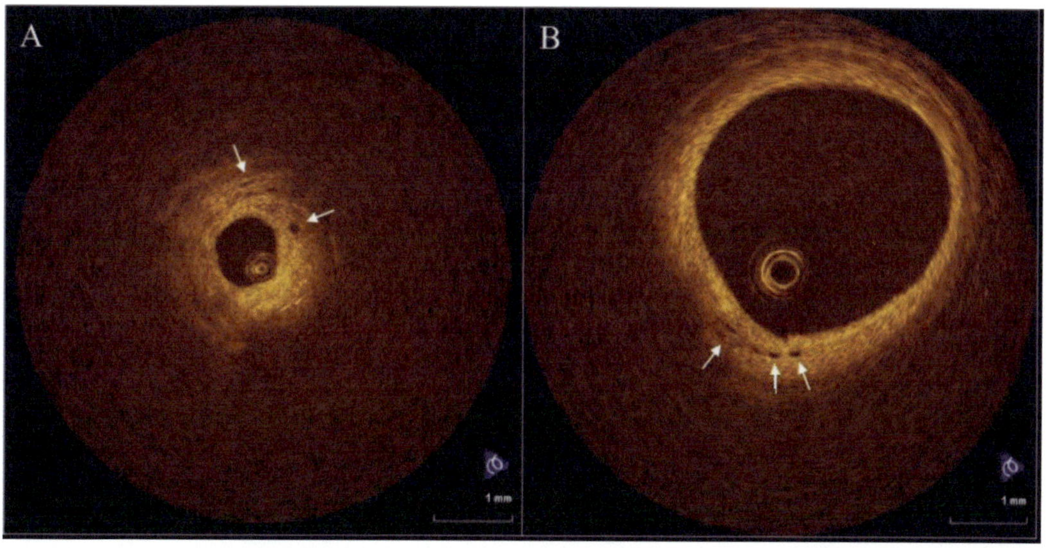

Figure 1. OCT (M2 system) images of plaque neovessels. Microvessels in the outer plaque (A) near the adventitia and (B) within the thickened intima can appear as signal-poor voids (white arrows) that are sharply delineated.

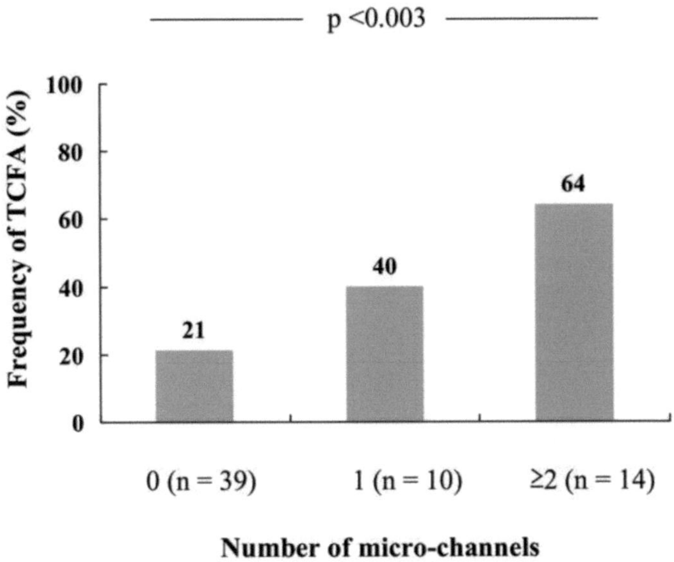

Figure 2. Comparison of frequency of TCFA according to number of microchannels. When categorized into 3 groups according to number of microchannels, the frequency of TCFA (21% in group with 0, 40% in group with 1, and 64% in group with ≥ 2; $p < 0.003$ for all) was significantly different. Reproduced with permission from [21].

5. Neovascularization inside the implanted stent by OCT

Although neovascularization within the neointima after stent implantation has been already reported in histopathologic studies [27, 28], Regar et al first reported in 2005 that OCT has an ability to visualize microvessels within the neointima inside the stents in a living human [29]. Later the presence of neovascularization in the stent restenosis was noted by Gonzalo et al [30]. However, the role of microvessels in restenotic tissue behavior has been unknown. More recently, Kim et al evaluated the characteristics of in-stent restenosis (ISR) lesions with microvessels detected by OCT [31]. Microvessels were detected in 21 (27%) of 78 ISR lesions. At the minimum lumen area site, the neointimal area (5.4 ± 1.7 mm^2 vs. 4.2 ± 2.1 mm^2, $p=0.024$) and percent neointimal area (79±12% vs. 67±16%, $p=0.001$) were significantly greater in ISR lesions with microvessels. These results suggest that microvessels within the neointima might be associated with restenosis by the excessive neointimal growth following stent implantation.

Furthermore, it has been shown that neointima in both BMS and DES can transform into atherosclerotic tissue with time although it occurs earlier in DES than BMS and that neoathrosclerosis progression inside the implanted stents may be associated with very late coronary events such as very late stent thrombosis after BMS and DES implantation [28, 32-40]. Using OCT, Takano et al examined the differences in neointima between early phase (< 6 months) and late phase (≥ 5 years) [35]. When compared with normal neointima proliferated

http://dx.doi.org/10.5772/53051

homogeneously in the early phase, neointima inside the BMS ≥ 5 years after implantation was characterized by marked signal attenuation and a diffuse border, suggesting lipid-laden intima. Its frequency was 67% and lipid-laden intima was not observed in the early phase. TCFA-like intima was also found in 29% of the patients in the late phase. Intimal disruption and thrombus were observed more frequently in the late phase as compared with the early phase (38% vs. 0% and 52% vs. 5%, respectively; $p < 0.05$). Notably, although there was no significant difference in terms of the incidence of peristent neovascularization (Figure 3A) between the 2 phases (81% vs. 60%, p=0.14), intraintima neovascularization (Figure 3B) was seen more frequently in the late phase than in the early phase (62% vs. 0%, $p < 0.01$) and in segments with lipid-laden intima than those in without lipid-laden intima (79% vs. 29%, p=0.026). Moreover, Habara et al evaluated the difference of tissue characteristics between early (within the first year) and very late (> 5 years, without restenosis within the first years) restenostic lesions after BMS implantation by using OCT [39]. There was a significant difference in the morphological characteristics of restenostic tissue between very late ISR (characterized by heterogeneous intima) and early ISR (characterized by homogeneous intima). Intraintima microvessels were observed only in the very late ISR group (16.3% vs. 0%, p=0.01). Thus, expansion of neovascularization from persistent to intraintimal area with time may contribute to atherosclerosis progression of neointima, as well as intra-plaque neovascularization of nonstent segments in native coronary arteries.

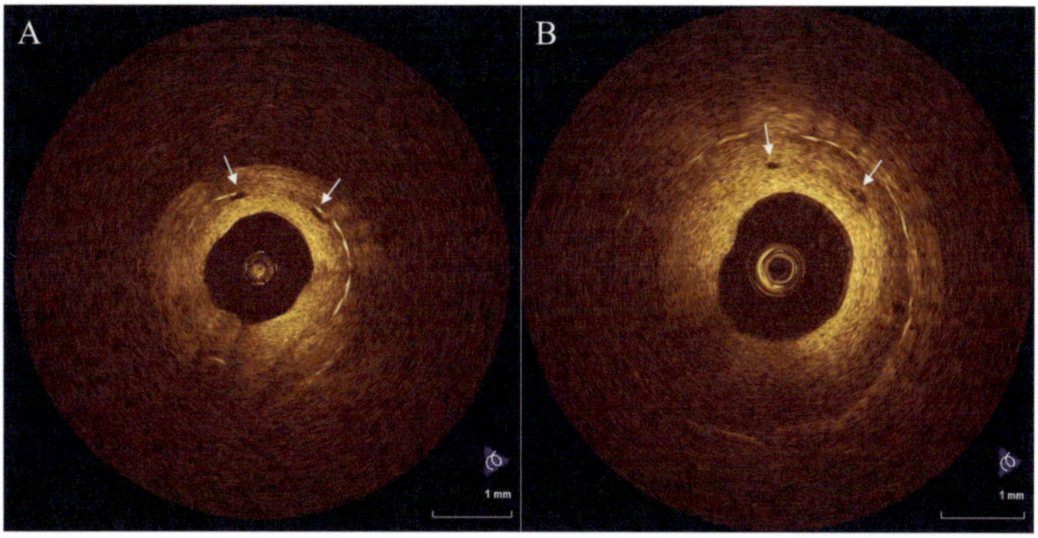

Figure 3. Neovascularization within neointima inside the implanted stent. (A) OCT (M2 system) image of peristent microvessels (arrows) demonstrating no-signal small vesicular and tubular structures locating around the struts. (B) OCT (M2 system) image of intraintima microvessels (arrows) showing small black holes locating near the vessel lumen within the neotintimal tissue.

6. Future perspectives (neovascularization as a therapeutic target for plaque stabilization)

For all cardiologists, stabilizing vulnerable plaques remains a major concern. Previous clinical trials have demonstrated that lipid-lowering therapy by statins stabilizes vulnerable plaques, thereby preventing cardiac events. Experimental studies have also shown that anti-atherosclerotic therapies can reduce plaque neovascularization [41-43] and that the inhibition of plaque neovascularization reduces progression of advanced atherosclerosis [41, 42]. Therefore, monitoring treatment effects of anti-atherosclerotic drugs using reliable surrogate markers may be useful to appropriately manage the patients. The thickness of fibrous cap in coronary plaque is a major determinant of plaque destabilization [44]. We recently reported that statins increased the fibrous cap thickness of plaques as assessed by OCT, indicating plaque stabilization [45, 46]. More recently, Tian et al investigated whether there was a difference in the effects of statin therapy between lesions with and without neovascularization [47]. As a result, despite a comparable reduction in serum cholesterol levels, the fibrous cap thickening was smaller in lesions with neovascularization than those without neovascularization after 6 and 12 months of statin treatment, which suggests that a more aggressive anti-atherosclerotic therapy may be required in patients with plaque with neovascularization. Thus, OCT allows us to monitor the response to anti-atherosclerotic therapies such as statins, and micro-channels in plaques identified by OCT could become a therapeutic target for plaque stabilization as important as the thickness of fibrous cap (Figure 4).

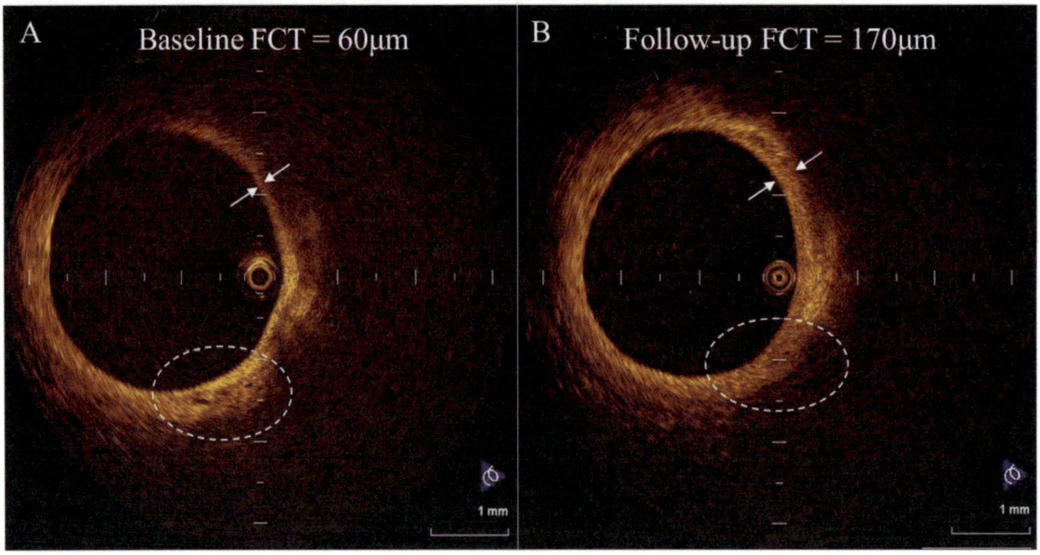

Figure 4. Plaque stabilization and elimination of neovascularization by statin treatment. (A) OCT (M2 system) demonstrates lipid-rich plaque covered by thin fibrous cap of 60 μm (thin-capped fibroatheroma) and microvessels at the shoulder region of the plaque (dotted circle). (B) Six months after statin treatment, the minimum fibrous cap thickness (FCT) increased from 60 μm to 170 μm and microvessels disappeared.

Moreover, a newer-generation Frequency-domain OCT (FD-OCT; C7 system, LightLab Imaging) has recently been developed to overcome many of the technical limitations of TD-OCT system by imaging at much higher frame rates (100 frame/s), a larger scan diameter (10 mm) and a faster image acquisition rate (20 mm/s) without loss of image quality, and unlike TD-OCT, this technology does not require proximal balloon occlusion [48]. The imaging catheter of FD-OCT, which is designed for rapid exchange delivery, has a 2.7-Fr crossing profile and can be delivered over a 0.014-inch guidewire through a 6-Fr or larger guide catheter. Intracoronary injection of contrast media via the guide catheter (3 to 4 ml/s; 2-3 s) can achieve effective clearing of blood for the FD-OCT imaging. In combination with a short, nonocclusive flush and a faster pullback speed, the FD-OCT enables imaging of longer segments of coronary arteries without significant ischemia and motion artifact [49]. Thus, we would be able to more precisely and easily assess not only culprit but also nonculprit lesion morphologies in coronary artery disease by use of FD-OCT.

7. Limitations

First, because the penetration depth of OCT is relatively shallow (<2 mm), and OCT light signals are limited behind the lipid component or red thrombus, previous OCT studies may underestimate the presence of neovascularization. Second, neovessel size has been inconsistently defined by a wide range because it is unknown whether there is a threshold for the size of these vessels within the intima [50]. Finally, a direct comparison of OCT-derived microchannels with histology has not been done to date. Therefore, histological studies that properly validate these structures observed with in vivo OCT imaging are mandatory in the near future.

8. Conclusions

OCT has the potential to directly visualize neovascularization of atherosclerotic plaques in vivo. Microchannel structure in coronary plaques identified by OCT could be a marker of plaque vulnerability to improve patient risk stratification and a therapeutic target for plaque stabilization.

Acknowledgement

The authors thank Takashi Kubo, MD; Kenichi Komukai, MD; Yasushi Ino, MD; Takashi Tanimoto, MD; Kohei Ishibashi, MD; Manabu Kashiwagi, MD; Yuichi Ozaki, MD; Kunihiro Shimamura, MD; Makoto Orii, MD; Yasutsugu Shiono, MD for assitance with OCT image acquisition and analysis.

Author details

Hironori Kitabata and Takashi Akasaka

Wakayama Medical University, Japan

References

[1] Boden WE, O'Rourke RA, Teo KK, Hartigan PM, Maron DJ, Kostuk WJ, Knudtson M, Dada M, Casperson P, Harris CL, Chaitman BR, Shaw L, Gosselin G, Nawaz S, Title LM, Gau G, Blaustein AS, Booth DC, Bates ER, Spertus JA, Berman DS, Mancini GB, Weintraub WS; COURAGE Trial Research Group. Optimal medical therapy with or without PCI for stable coronary disease. N Engl J Med 2007;356(15):1503-1516.

[2] Jeziorska M, Woolley DE. Neovascularization in early atherosclerotic lesions of human carotid arteries: its potential contribution to plaque development. Hum Pathol 1999;30(8):919-925.

[3] Barger AC, Beeuwkes R, Lainey L, Silverman KJ. Hypothesis: vasa vasorum and neovascularization of human coronary arteries. N Engl J Med 1984;310(3):175-177.

[4] Barger AC, Beeuwkes R. Rupture of coronary vasa vasorum as a trigger of acute myocardial infarction. Am J Cardiol 1990;66(16):41G-43G.

[5] Tenaglia AN, Peters KG, Sketch MH Jr, Annex BH. Neovascularization in atherectomy specimens from patients with unstable angina: implications for pathogenesis of unstable angina. Am Heart J 1998;135(1):10-14.

[6] Kume T, Akasaka T, Kawamoto T, Watanabe N, Toyota E, Sukmawan R, Sadahira Y, Yoshida K. Assessment of coronary arterial plaque by optical coherence tomography. Am J Cardiol 2006;97(8):1172–1175.

[7] Kume T, Akasaka T, Kawamoto T, Watanabe N, Toyota E, Neishi Y, Sukmawan R, Sadahira Y, Yoshida K. Assessment of coronary intima-media thickness by optical coherence tomography: comparison with intravascular ultrasound. Circ J 2005;69(8): 903-907.

[8] Yabushita H, Bouma BE, Houser SL, Aretz HT, Jang IK, Schlendorf KH, Kauffman CR, Shishkov M, Kang DH, Halpern EF, Tearney GJ. Characterization of human atherosclerosis by optical coherence tomography. Circulation 2002;106(13):1640-1645.

[9] Moreno PR, Purushothaman KR, Sirol M, Levy AP, Fuster V. Neovascularization in human atherosclerosis. Circulation 2006;113(18):2245-2252.

[10] Virmani R, Kolodgie FD, Burke AP, Finn AV, Gold HK, Tulenko TN, Wrenn SP, Narula J. Atherosclerotic plaque progression and vulnerability to rupture: angiogenesis

as a source of intraplaque hemorrhage. Arterioscler Thromb Vasc Biol. 2005;25(10): 2054-2061.

[11] Moreno PR, Purushothaman KR, Fuster V, Echeverri D, Truszczynska H, Sharma SK, Badimon JJ, O'Connor WN. Plaque neovascularization is increased in ruptured atherosclerotic lesions of human aorta: implications for plaque vulnerability. Circulation 2004;110(14):2032-2038.

[12] Herrmann J, Lerman LO, Rodriguez-Porcel M, Holmes DR Jr, Richardson DM, Ritman EL, Lerman A. Coronary vasa vasorum neovascularization precedes epicardial endothelial dysfunction in experimental hypercholesterolemia. Cardiovasc Res 2001;51(4):762-766.

[13] Gössl M, Versari D, Mannheim D, Ritman EL, Lerman LO, Lerman A. Increased spatial vasa vasorum density in the proximal LAD in hypercholesterolemia; implications for vulnerable plaque-development. Atherosclerosis 2007;192(2):246-252.

[14] Winter PM, Morawski AM, Caruthers SD, Fuhrhop RW, Zhang H, Williams TA, Allen JS, Lacy EK, Robertson JD, Lanza GM, Wickline SA. Molecular imaging of angiogenesis in early-stage atherosclerosis with alpha (v) beta3-integrin-targeted nanoparticles. Circulation 2003;108(18):2270-2274.

[15] Sirol M, Moreno PR, Purushothaman KR, Vucic E, Amirbekian V, Weinmann HJ, Muntner P, Fuster V, Fayad ZA. Increased neovascularization in advanced lipid-rich atherosclerotic lesions detected by gadofluorine-M-enhanced MRI: implications for plaque vulnerability. Circ Cardiovasc Imaging. 2009;2(5):391-396.

[16] Vavuranakis M, Kakadiaris IA, O'Malley SM, Papaioannou TG, Sanidas EA, Naghavi M, Carlier S, Tousoulis D, Stefanadis C. A new method for assessment of plaque vulnerability based on vasa vasorum imaging, by using contrast-enhanced intravascular ultrasound and differential image analysis. Int J Cardiol 2008;130(1):23-29.

[17] Granada JF, Feinstein SB. Imaging of the vasa vasorum. Nat Clin Pract Cardiovasc Med 2008;5 Suppl 2:S18-25.

[18] Kubo T, Imanishi T, Takarada S, Kuroi A, Ueno S, Yamano T, Tanimoto T, Matsuo Y, Masho T, Kitabata H, Tsuda K, Tomobuchi Y, Akasaka T. Assessment of culprit lesion morphology in acute myocardial infarction: ability of optical coherence tomography compared with intravascular ultrasound and coronary angioscopy. J Am Coll Cardiol 2007;50(10):933-939.

[19] Jang IK, Tearney GJ, MacNeill B, Takano M, Moselewski F, Iftima N, Shishkov M, Houser S, Aretz HT, Halpern EF, Bouma BE. In vivo characterization of coronary atherosclerotic plaque by use of optical coherence tomography. Circulation 2005;111(12):1551-1555.

[20] Prati F, Regar E, Mintz GS, Arbustini E, Di Mario C, Jang IK, Akasaka T, Costa M, Guagliumi G, Grube E, Ozaki Y, Pinto F, Serruys PW; for the Expert's OCT Review Document. Expert review document on methodology, terminology, and clinical ap-

plications of optical coherence tomography: physical principles, methodology of image acquisition, and clinical application for assessment of coronary arteries and atherosclerosis. Eur Heart J 2009;31(4):401-415.

[21] Kitabata H, Tanaka A, Kubo T, Takarada S, Kashiwagi M, Tsujioka H, Ikejima H, Kuroi A, Kataiwa H, Ishibashi K, Komukai K, Tanimoto T, Ino Y, Hirata K, Nakamura N, Mizukoshi M, Imanishi T, Akasaka T. Relation of microchannel structure identified by optical coherence tomography to plaque vulnerability in patients with coronary artery disease. Am J Cardiol 2010;105(12):1673-1678.

[22] Tian J, Hou J, Xing L, Kim SJ, Yonetsu T, Kato K, Lee H, Zhang S, Yu B, Jang IK. Significance of intraplaque neovascularisation for vulnerability: optical coherence tomography study. Heart 2012 Aug 6. [Epub ahead of print]

[23] Kato K, Yonetsu T, Kim SJ, Xing L, Lee H, McNulty I, Yeh RW, Sakhuja R, Zhang S, Uemura S, Yu B, Mizuno K, Jang IK. Nonculprit plaques in patients with acute coronary syndromes have more vulnerable features compared with those with non-acute coronary syndromes: a 3-vessel optical coherence tomography study. Circ Cardiovasc Imaging 2012;5(4):433-440.

[24] Uemura S, Ishigami K, Soeda T, Okayama S, Sung JH, Nakagawa H, Somekawa S, Takeda Y, Kawata H, Horii M, Saito Y. Thin-cap fibroatheroma and microchannel findings in optical coherence tomography correlate with subsequent progression of coronary atheromatous plaques. Eur Heart J. 2012;33(1):78-85.

[25] Vorpahl M, Nakano M, Virmani R. Small black holes in optical frequency domain imaging matches intravascular neoangiogenesis formation in histology. Eur Heart J 2010;31(15):1889.

[26] Kumamoto M, Nakashima Y, Sueishi K. Intimal neovascularization in human coronary atherosclerosis: its origin and pathophysiological significance. Hum Pathol 1995;26(4):450-456.

[27] Komatsu R, Ueda M, Naruko T, Kojima A, Becker AE. Neointimal tissue response at sites of coronary stenting in humans: macroscopic, histological, and immunohistochemical analyses. Circulation 1998;98(3):224-233.

[28] Inoue K, Abe K, Ando K, Shirai S, Nishiyama K, Nakanishi M, Yamada T, Sakai K, Nakagawa Y, Hamasaki N, Kimura T, Nobuyoshi M, Miyamoto TA. Pathological analyses of long-term intracoronary Palmaz-Schatz stenting; Is its efficacy permanent? Cardiovasc Pathol 2004;13(2):109-115.

[29] Regar E, van Beusekom HMM, van der Gissen WJ, Serruys PW. Optical coherence tomography findings at 5-year follow-up after coronary stent implantation. Circulation 2005;112(23):e345–e346.

[30] Gonzalo N, Serruys PW, Okamura T, van Beusekom HM, Garcia-Garcia HM, van Soest G, van der Giessen W, Regar E. Optical coherence tomography patterns of stent restenosis. Am Heart J 2009;158(2):284-93.

[31] Kim BK, Kim JS, Shin DH, Ko YG, Choi D, Jang Y, Hong MK. Optical coherence tomography evaluation of in-stent restenotic lesions with visible microvessels. J Invasive Cardiol 2012;24(3):116-20.

[32] Hasegawa K, Tamai H, Kyo E, Kosuga K, Ikeguchi S, Hata T, Okada M, Fujita S, Tsuji T, Takeda S, Fukuhara R, Kikuta Y, Motohara S, Ono K, Takeuchi E. Histopathological findings of new in-stent lesions developed beyond five years. Catheter Cardiovasc Interv 2006;68(4):554-558.

[33] Yokoyama S, Takano M, Yamamoto M, Inami S, Sakai S, Okamatsu K, Okuni S, Seimiya K, Murakami D, Ohba T, Uemura R, Seino Y, Hata N, Mizuno K. Extended follow-up by serial angioscopic observation for bare-metal stents in native coronary arteries: from healing response to atherosclerotic transformation of neointimal. Circ Cardiovasc Intervent 2009;2(3):205-212.

[34] Kashiwagi M, Kitabata H, Tanaka A, Okochi K, Ishibashi K, Komukai K, Tanimoto T, Ino Y, Takarada S, Kubo T, Hirata K, Mizukoshi M, Imanishi T, Akasaka T. Very late cardiac event after BMS implantation: In vivo optical coherence tomography examination. J Am Coll Cardiol Img 2010;3(5):525-527.

[35] Takano M, Yamamoto M, Inami S, Murakami D, Ohba T, Seino Y, Mizuno K. Appearance of lipid-laden intima and neovascularization after implantation of bare-metal stents. J Am Coll Cardiol 2010;55(1):26-32.

[36] Hou J, Qi H, Zhang M, Ma L, Liu H, Han Z, Meng L, Yang S, Zhang S, Yu B, Jang IK. Development of lipid-rich plaque inside bare metal stent: possible mechanism of late stent thrombosis? An optical coherence tomography study. Heart 2010;96(15): 1187-90.

[37] Nakazawa G, Otsuka F, Nakano M, Vorpahl M, Yazdani SK, Ladich E, Kolodgie FD, Finn AV, Virmani R. The pathology of neoatherosclerosis in human coronary implants: bare-metal and drug-eluting stents. J Am Coll Cardiol 2011;57(11):1314-1322.

[38] Kang SJ, Mintz GS, Akasaka T, Park DW, Lee JY, Kim WJ, Lee SW, Kim YH, Whan Lee C, Park SW, Park SJ. Optical coherence tomographic analysis of in-stent neoatherosclerosis after drug-eluting stent implantation. Circulation 2011;123(25): 2954-2963.

[39] Habara M, Terashima M, Nasu K, Kaneda H, Inoue K, Ito T, Kamikawa S, Kurita T, Tanaka N, Kimura M, Kinoshita Y, Tsuchikane E, Matsuo H, Ueno K, Katoh O, Suzuki T. Difference of tissue characteristics between early and very late restenosis lesions after bare-metal stent implantation: an optical coherence tomography study. Circ Cardiovasc Interv 2011;4(3):232-238

[40] Kitabata H, Kubo T, Komukai K, Ishibashi K, Tanimoto T, Ino Y, Takarada S, Ozaki Y, Kashiwagi M, Orii M, Shiono M, Shimamura K, Hirata K, Tanaka A, Kimura K, Mizukoshi M, Imanishi T, Akasaka T. Effect of strut thickness on neointimal atherosclerotic change over an extended follow-up period (≥ 4 years) after bare-metal stent

implantation: intracoronary optical coherence tomography examination. Am Heart J 2012;163(4):608-616.

[41] Moulton KS, Heller E, Konerding MA, Flynn E, Palinski W, Folkman J. Angiogenesis inhibitors endostatin or TNP-470 reduce intimal neovascularization and plaque growth in apolipoprotein E-deficient mice. Circulation 1999;99(13):1726-1732.

[42] Moulton KS, Vakili K, Zurakowski D, Soliman M, Butterfield C, Sylvin E, Lo KM, Gillies S, Javaherian K, Folkman J. Inhibition of plaque neovascularization reduces macrophage accumulation and progression of advanced atherosclerosis. Proc Natl Acad Sci U S A 2003;100(8):4736-4741.

[43] Wilson SH, Herrmann J, Lerman LO, Holmes DR, Napoli C, Ritman EL, Lerman A. Simvastatin preserves the structure of coronary adventitial vasa vasorum in experimental hypercholesterolemia independent of lipid lowering. Circulation 2002;105(4): 415-418.

[44] Virmani R, Kolodgie FD, Burke AP, Farb A, Schwartz SM. Lessons from sudden coronary death: a comprehensive morphological classification scheme for atherosclerotic lesions. Arterioscler Thromb Vasc Bio 2000;20(5):1262-1275.

[45] Takarada S, Imanishi T, Kubo T, Tanimoto T, Kitabata H, Nakamura N, Tanaka A, Mizukoshi M, Akasaka T. Effect of statin therapy on coronary fibrous-cap thickness in patients with acute coronary syndrome: Assessment by optical coherence tomography study. Atherosclerosis 2009;202(2):491-497.

[46] Takarada S, Imanishi T, Ishibashi K, Tanimoto T, Komukai K, Ino Y, Kitabata H, Kubo T, Tanaka A, Kimura K, Mizukoshi M, Akasaka T. The effect of lipid and inflammatory profiles on the morphological changes of lipid-rich plaques in patients with non-ST-segment elevated acute coronary syndrome: follow-up study by optical coherence tomography and intravascular ultrasound. J Am Coll Cardiol Intv 2010;3(7): 766-772.

[47] Tian J, Hou J, Xing L, Kim SJ, Yonetsu T, Kato K, Lee H, Zhang S, Yu B, Jang IK. Does neovascularization predict response to statin therapy? Optical coherence tomography study. Int J Cardiol 2012;158(3):469-470.

[48] Barlis P, Schmitt JM: Current and future developments in intracoronary optical coherence tomography imaging. EuroIntervention 2009;4(4):529-533.

[49] Takarada S, Imanishi T, Liu Y, Ikejima H, Tsujioka H, Kuroi A, Ishibashi K, Komukai K, Tanimoto T, Ino Y, Kitabata H, Kubo T, Nakamura N, Hirata K, Tanaka A, Mizukoshi M, Akasaka T. Advantage of next-generation frequency domain optical coherence tomography compared with conventional time-domain system in the assessment of coronary lesion. Catheter Cardiovasc Interv 2010;75(2):202-206.

[50] Tearney GJ, Regar E, Akasaka T, Adriaenssens T, Barlis P, Bezerra HG, Bouma B, Bruining N, Cho JM, Chowdhary S, Costa MA, de Silva R, Dijkstra J, Di Mario C, Dudek D, Falk E, Feldman MD, Fitzgerald P, Garcia-Garcia HM, Gonzalo N, Granada

JF, Guagliumi G, Holm NR, Honda Y, Ikeno F, Kawasaki M, Kochman J, Koltowski L, Kubo T, Kume T, Kyono H, Lam CC, Lamouche G, Lee DP, Leon MB, Maehara A, Manfrini O, Mintz GS, Mizuno K, Morel MA, Nadkarni S, Okura H, Otake H, Pietrasik A, Prati F, Räber L, Radu MD, Rieber J, Riga M, Rollins A, Rosenberg M, Sirbu V, Serruys PW, Shimada K, Shinke T, Shite J, Siegel E, Sonoda S, Suter M, Takarada S, Tanaka A, Terashima M, Thim T, Uemura S, Ughi GJ, van Beusekom HM, van der Steen AF, van Es GA, van Soest G, Virmani R, Waxman S, Weissman NJ, Weisz G; International Working Group for Intravascular Optical Coherence Tomography (IWG-IVOCT).Consensus standards for acquisition, measurement, and reporting of intravascular optical coherence tomography studies: a report from the International Working Group for Intravascular Optical Coherence Tomography Standardization and Validation. J Am Coll Cardiol 2012;59(12):1058-1072.

Chapter 6

Optical Coherence Tomography (OCT): A New Imaging Tool During Carotid Artery Stenting

Shinichi Yoshimura, Masanori Kawasaki, Kiyofumi Yamada, Arihiro Hattori, Kazuhiko Nishigaki, Shinya Minatoguchi and Toru Iwama

Additional information is available at the end of the chapter

http://dx.doi.org/10.5772/53962

1. Introduction

One of the mechanisms underlying acute stroke is the disruption of atherosclerotic plaques in major cerebral vessels, including the carotid arteries. However, visualizing precise arterial wall changes is sometimes difficult using conventional imaging techniques such as angiography, magnetic resonance imaging (MRI) or duplex ultrasonography. In particular, intraluminal thrombus is difficult to detect clearly during catheter interventions such as carotid artery stenting (CAS), even with utilization of intravascular ultrasonography (IVUS) [1,2]. When visualization of the carotid wall changes is possible during CAS, especially before and after angioplasty and stenting, it then becomes possible be to select appropriate devices and methods of angioplasty and cerebral protection based on better anatomical information.

Intravascular optical coherence tomography (OCT) has recently been proposed as a high-resolution imaging tool for plaque characterization in the coronary arteries. OCT is a non-contact, light-based imaging method utilizing newly developed fiber-optic technology (Fig. 1). The typical OCT image has an axial resolution of 10 μm, approximately 10 times higher than that of any other clinically available diagnostic imaging modality such as IVUS with a resolution of 80 μm [3]. Therefore, despite the need for removing blood from the field of view, in vivo application of OCT has been reported useful in the coronary arteries [4-7]. For example, Jang IK et al reported that intracoronary OCT identified most architectural features detected by IVUS and provided additional detailed structural information [4]. Kawasaki M et al claimed that OCT had the best potential for tissue characterization of coronary plaques, within the penetration depth of OCT, in a comparative study with IVUS [7]. Based on these results, we speculated that intravascular OCT would also be useful for the other vessels. Our use of OCT for human carotid arteries was approved by our institutional review board (No. 21-108), and recently registered on the Internet (University Hospital Medical Information Network: UMIN 000002808).

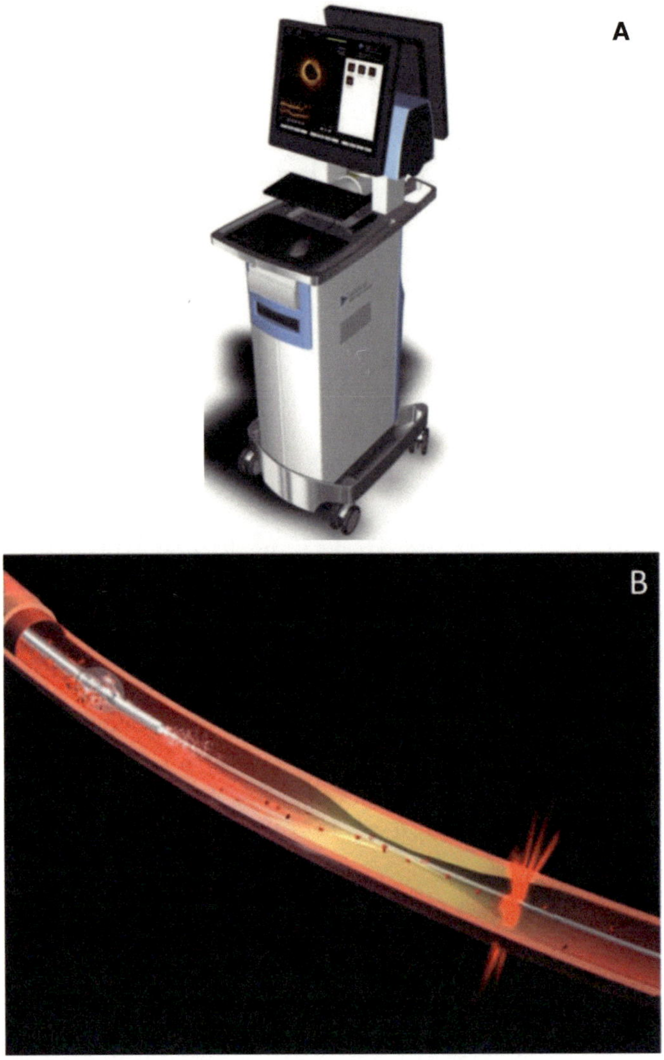

Figure 1. Images of an optical coherence tomography (OCT) system and an imagewire. This is the first generation of OCT analyzer (M2 OCT Imaging system, LightLab Imaging, Inc., Westford, Massachusetts, A), which was used for our clinical studies. An imagewire is schematically demonstrated to show its scanning capabilities during the target artery occlusion using an occlusion balloon (B).

2. First application of OCT for the human carotid artery

Our group first applied intravascular OCT in a patient with a large thrombus in the carotid artery [8]. An 83-year old male admitted due to motor weakness of the left hand. Diffusion weighted MRI showed multiple high intensity spots in the territory of the right middle cerebral artery, and magnetic resonance angiography (MRA) revealed significant stenosis at the origin of the right internal carotid artery (Fig. 2A). Because of an apparent change in plaque shape on the angiogram just before CAS (Fig. 2B), further examinations such as IVUS and OCT were performed. After IVUS examination (Fig. 2D), both the common carotid and external carotid arteries were occluded by an occlusion balloon system prepared for CAS. Then, the stenotic site was imaged by OCT (M2 OCT Imaging system, LightLab Imaging, Inc., Westford, Massachusetts) from the distal section at 1mm/sec using a built-in pull-back system with continuous injection of saline through the guiding catheter to remove blood from the field of view. Intraluminal thrombus was clearly demonstrated by OCT (Fig. 2C), and carotid endarterectomy was performed instead of stenting to avoid distal migration of the thrombus during the revascularization procedure. The carotid artery specimen obtained by endarterectomy showed a soft plaque with a large intraluminal thrombus, which correlated with OCT findings performed preoperatively (Fig. 2E,F). This was the first report of a clinical application of the OCT in the carotid artery, and the intraluminal thrombus detected by OCT was successfully confirmed by histological analysis of the surgical specimen.

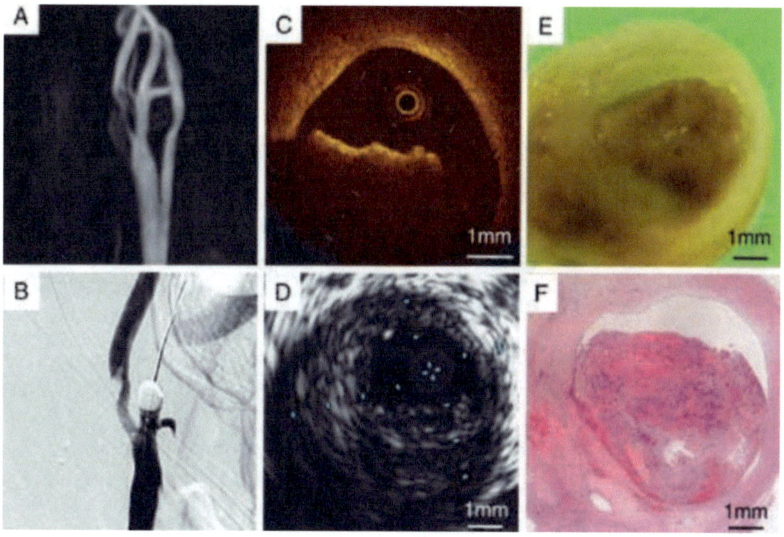

Figure 2. An intraluminal thrombus in the carotid artery demonstrated by OCT and confirmed by pathological analysis.A: initial magnetic resonance angiography revealed severe stenosis of the internal carotid artery (ICA) and high-intensity plaque. B: the carotid angiogram showed ICA stenosis and enlargement of an intraluminal protrusion in the ICA. C: cross sections by OCT demonstrated an intraluminal thrombus with shadowing in the ICA. D: cross sections by intravascular ultrasonography showed only eccentric and low-echoic plaque in the ICA.E: macroscopic view of a surgical specimen showing an intraluminal thrombus formed at the ruptured site of the plaque. F: pathological analysis with hematoxylin-eosin staining confirmed soft plaque with intraplaque hemorrhage and an intraluminal red thrombus, which correlated with OCT findings. This study was reported previously [8].

It has been reported that neither angiography nor IVUS can reliably demonstrate the presence of a thrombus [1]. In this patient, a thrombus in the carotid artery was clearly demonstrated by preoperative OCT. Due to the size of thrombus the information provided by OCT which altered therapy, possible embolism and its consequences of hemiparesis or speech disturbance was averted.

Kume et al reported that OCT could differentiate between red and white coronary arterial thrombi by post mortem, ex vivo experiments [9]. Meng et al reported on the feasibility of OCT for the detection of in vivo acute thrombosis in the carotid artery using an animal model [10]. They also reported an excellent correlation between OCT images and histology regarding thrombus length and location. OCT images of red thrombi are characterized as highly backscattered protrusions with signal-free shadowing. A red thrombus consists mainly of red blood cells, causing scatter and attenuation of OCT signal intensity from the inner surface of the thrombus to the vessel wall. In our patient, the protruded mass in the ICA (Fig. 2B) was diagnosed as a red thrombus by OCT (Fig. 2C) because of signal attenuation behind the mass, and pathologically confirmed thereafter (Fig. 2E,F).

3. Comparison of OCT with IVUS during stenting

Next, this group applied OCT for the carotid artery during stenting as a clinical study. In this study, we evaluated the ability of OCT to visualize structures of the carotid artery wall when compared with IVUS. We reported typical images of this preliminary OCT application to human carotid arteries during CAS [11]. OCT was performed on 20 plaques of 17 patients

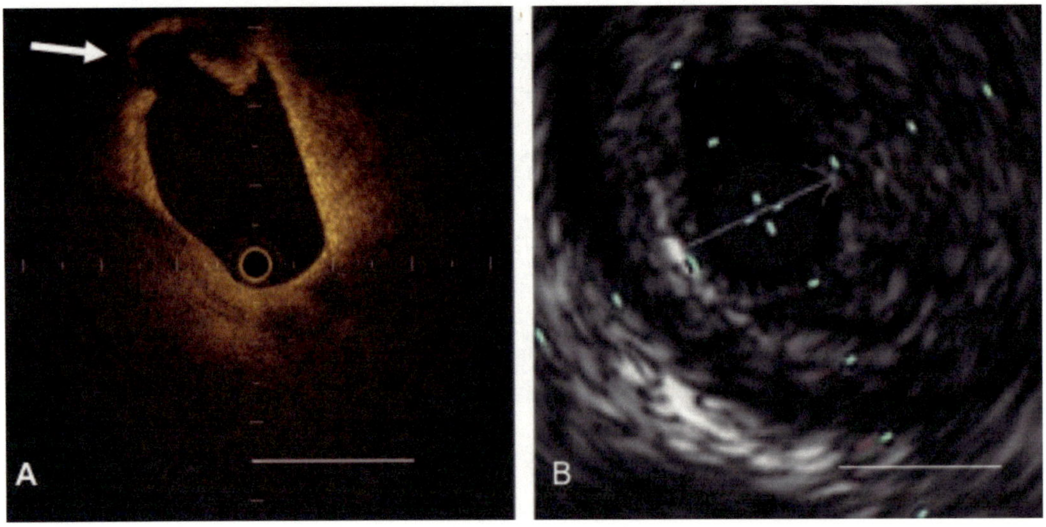

Figure 3. Representative images of carotid plaque with fibrous cap disruption from a symptomatic patient with right ICA stenosis prior to carotid artery stenting (CAS). A: an image from OCT shows fibrous cap disruption as a discontinuous fibrous cap and cavity formation (arrow). B: IVUS was not able to detect the fibrous cap disruption. The bar in both A and B equals 2 mm. This study was reported previously [11].

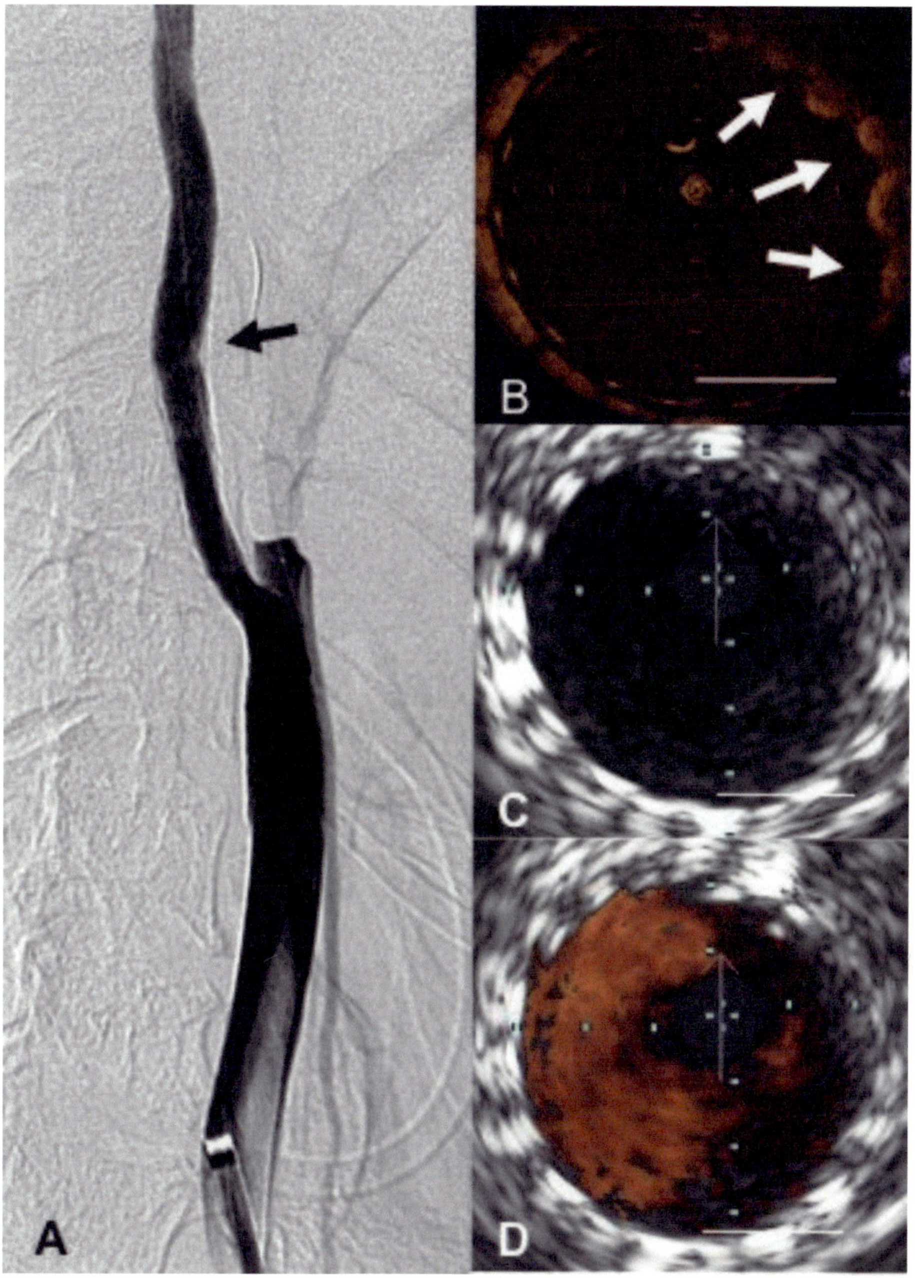

Figure 4. Tissue Protrusion. Representative images of carotid plaque protrusion in a symptomatic patient with left ICA stenosis after carotid artery stenting (CAS). Plaque protrusion is considered to be one source for the embolic complication after CAS. Plaque protrusion from stent struts just after stent deployment was clearly demonstrated by OCT, but was overlooked by IVUS. A: Carotid angiogram demonstrating the plaque protrusion after stent placement (arrow). B: OCT demonstrates tissue protrusion from spaces between stent struts (white arrows). C, D: IVUS with and without ChromaFlo (Eagle Eye Gold, Volcano Therapeutics, Rancho Cordova, California) was unable to see plaque protrusions. The bar in B, C, and D equals 2 mm. This study was reported previously [11].

during CAS, under a proximal cerebral protection method. In addition to intraluminal thrombus, fibrous cap disruption (Fig. 3) and plaque protrusion after stenting (Fig. 4) were easily detected by OCT. There were no technical or neurological complications in this series. OCT could best visualize the lateral side of lumen pathology (intraluminal thrombus or fibrous cap disruption) with a high resolution of 10 um, whereas IVUS, MRI, or computed tomography allowed assessment of the entire arterial wall, albeit with lesser resolution. OCT and IVUS thus complement each other and may aid in discriminating plaques that are eligible for CAS.

4. Differences between symptomatic and asymptomatic plaques by OCT

Another study to evaluate the ability of OCT to visualize carotid artery plaques as compared to that of IVUS in asymptomatic and symptomatic patients was performed [12]. In this study, OCT was used for 34 plaques (17 symptomatic, 17 asymptomatic) in 30 patients during CAS under a proximal cerebral protection method. OCT was performed before balloon angioplasty and after stent placement. IVUS was performed after OCT. Among pre-stenting findings, intraluminal thrombus and neovascularization were significantly more frequently detected by OCT than by VH-IVUS ($p<0.001$). Ulceration also tended to be more frequently detected by OCT than by IVUS, but the difference was not significant (Table 1). Conversely, calcification was less frequently detected by OCT than by IVUS ($p<0.001$; Table 1). No difference in the detection of the lipid rich necrotic core was seen between OCT and IVUS (Table 1).

	OCT	VH-IVUS	p-value
Pre-stenting (n = 34)			
Thrombus, n (%)	15 (44.1)	1 (2.9)	<0.001
Neovascularization, n (%)	13 (38.2)	0 (0)	<0.001
Ulceration, n (%)	3 (8.8)	0 (0)	0.24
Calcification, n (%)	13 (38.2)	34 (100)*	<0.001
Lipid, n (%)	28 (82.4)	30 (88.2)**	0.73
Post-stenting (n = 34)			
Plaque protrusion, n (%)	6 (17.6)	0 (0)	0.032

*: shown as 'dense calcified', **: shown as 'fibrofatty and/or necrotic core' on VH-IVUS

Table 1. Comparison of OCT and VH-IVUS findings

OCT detected differences between symptomatic and asymptomatic carotid plaques (Table 2): intraluminal thrombus was more frequently observed in symptomatic plaques (76.5%) than in asymptomatic plaques (11.8%; $p<0.001$); and, neovascularization was also more often observed in symptomatic plaques (58.8%) than in asymptomatic plaques (17.6%; $p=0.03$). In contrast, no significant differences were seen in the incidence of other findings such as

http://dx.doi.org/10.5772/53962

calcification, lipid-rich necrotic core, ulceration, and plaque protrusion after stent placement between groups. *Interobserver* and intraobserver variability with OCT diagnosis was excellent for thrombus, ulceration, neovascularization, and lipid pool.

	Symptomatic	**Asymptomatic**	**p-value**
	(n=17)	**(n=17)**	
Male, n (%)	14 (82.4)	15 (88.2)	"/>0.99
Age, yr	72 ± 10	68 ± 10	0.19
Degree of stenosis, %	84 ± 12	79 ± 7	0.26
OCT findings			
Thrombus	13 (76.5)	2 (11.8)	<0.001
Neovascularization	10 (58.8)	3 (17.6)	0.03
Ulceration	3 (17.6)	0 (0)	0.23
Calcification	7 (41.2)	6 (35.3)	"/>0.99
Lipid-rich component	16 (94.1)	12 (70.6)	0.17
Plaque protrusion	4 (23.5)	2 (11.8)	0.66

Table 2. OCT findings of symptomatic and asymptomatic lesions

5. Limitations and recent advances of the OCT system

The major limitations of OCT are interference by blood flow and the degree of tissue penetration. To obtain a bloodless field of view, a proximal protection method which uses occlusion balloons for the common and external carotid arteries is required for the application of OCT in the cervical carotid artery [8, 11, 12]. The scanning length of OCT was 3.25 to 3.4 mm in normal saline. Therefore, in the carotid artery, plaque components located on the far side of the luminal surface were sometimes not visualized by OCT due to its limited penetration depth. Recently, a new frequency domain OCT system was developed. This new system does not need occlusion of the target artery due to faster scanning (Table 3). Setacci et al. document the benefits of this new OCT system utilizing a non-occlusive technique in the carotid artery [13]. In their report, the new system not only safely eliminated the need to occlude the carotid artery, but also acquired good quality images and informative details before and after stenting. Notably, the new OCT catheter can visualize arteries up to 10 mm in diameter, encompassing the entire carotid artery. Thus, this new system seems to overcome the imitations of the previous iteration, allowing OCT to be applied safely, easily, and efficiently in the carotid artery. Future studies are expected to investigate the relationship between carotid plaques and stents with regard to stent design and plaque composition.

	New version (C7)	Previous version (M2)
Axial Resolution	12 - 15 • m	15 - 20 • m
Beam Width	20 – 40 • m	20 – 40 • m
Frame Rate	100 frames/s	15 frames/s
Pullback Speed	20 mm/s	2 mm/s
Max. Scan Dia.	10 mm	6.8 mm
Tissue Penetration	1.0 - 2.0 mm	1.0 - 2.0 mm
Lines per Frame	500	200
Lateral Resolution (3mm Artery)	19 • m	39 • m

Table 3. Comparison of new and previous version of OCT

6. Conclusions

Optical coherence tomography (OCT) is a useful tool in the assessment of intraluminal thrombus before interventional procedure. Also, its excellent resolution may detect plaque protrusions after carotid artery stenting alerting to possible complications. Further studies with a new system utilizing a non-occlusive technique are expected to investigate the clinical applicability of OCT to characterize carotid plaque components and intraluminal changes during CAS.

Acknowledgements

We have no financial or other relations that could lead to a conflict of interest.

Author details

Shinichi Yoshimura[1*], Masanori Kawasaki[2], Kiyofumi Yamada[2], Arihiro Hattori[2], Kazuhiko Nishigaki[2], Shinya Minatoguchi[1] and Toru Iwama[1]

*Address all correspondence to: shinichiyoshimura@hotmail.com

1 Department of Neurosurgery, and Regeneration & Advanced Medical Science, Graduate School of Medicine, Gifu University, Gifu, Japan

2 Department of Radiology, University of Washington, Seattle, USA

References

[1] Timaran, C. H, Rosero, E. B, Martinez, A. E, et al. Atherosclerotic plaque composition assessed by virtual histology intravascular ultrasound and cerebral embolization after carotid stenting. J Vasc Surg (2010). , 52, 1188-94.

[2] Hishikawa, T, Iihara, K, Ishibashi-ueda, H, et al. Virtual histology-intravascular ultrasound in assessment of carotid plaques: ex vivo study. Neurosurgery (2009). , 65, 146-52.

[3] Mintz, G. S, Nissen, S. E, Anderson, W. D, et al. American College of Cardiology clinical expert consensus document on standards for acquisition, measurement and reporting of intravascular ultrasound studies (IVUS). A report of the American College of Cardiology task force on clinical expert consensus documents developed in collaboration with the European society of cardiology endorsed by the society of cardiac angiography and interventions. J Am Coll Cardiol (2001). , 37, 1478-92.

[4] Jang, I. K, Bouma, B. E, Kang, D. H, et al. Visualization of coronary atherosclerotic plaques in patients using optical coherence tomography: comparison with intravascular ultrasound. J Am Coll Cardiol (2002). , 39, 604-9.

[5] Yabushita, H, Bouma, B. E, Houser, S. L, et al. Characterization of human atherosclerosis by optical coherence tomography. Circulation (2002). , 106, 1640-5.

[6] Jang, I. K, & Tearney, G. J. MacNeill B, et al. In vivo characterization of coronary atherosclerotic plaque by use of optical coherence tomography. Circulation (2005). , 111, 1551-5.

[7] Kawasaki, M, Bouma, B. E, Bressner, J, et al. Diagnostic accuracy of optical coherence tomography and integrated backscatter intravascular ultrasound images for tissue characterization of human coronary plaques. J Am Coll Cardiol (2006). , 48, 81-8.

[8] Yoshimura, S, Kawasaki, M, Yamada, K, et al. Demonstration of intraluminal thrombus in the carotid artery by optical coherence tomography. Neurosurgery (2010). Suppl Operative):onsE305.

[9] Kume, T, Akasaka, T, Kawamoto, T, et al. Assessment of coronary arterial thrombus by optical coherence tomography. Am J Cardiol (2006). , 97, 1713-7.

[10] Meng, L, Lv, B, Zhang, S, & Yv, B. In vivo optical coherence tomography of experimental thrombosis in a rabbit carotid model. Heart (2008). , 94, 777-80.

[11] Yoshimura, S, Kawasaki, M, Yamada, K, et al. OCT of human carotid arterial plaques. JACC Cardiovasc Imaging (2011). , 4, 432-6.

[12] Yoshimura, S, Kawasaki, M, Yamada, K, et al. Visualization of internal carotid artery atherosclerotic plaques in symptomatic and asymptomatic patients: a comparison of optical coherence tomography and intravascular ultrasound. AJNR Am J Neuroradiol (2012). , 33, 308-13.

[13] Setacci, C, De Donato, G, Setacci, F, et al. Safety and feasibility of intravascular optical coherence tomography using a nonocclusive technique to evaluate carotid plaques before and after stent deployment. J Endovasc Ther (2012). , 19, 303-11.

[14] Yoshimura, S. Intravascular optical coherence tomography: a new, more detailed view of the carotid arteries. J Endovasc Ther (2012). , 19, 314-5.

Chapter 7

Optical Coherence Tomography for Coronary Artery Plaques – A Comparison with Intravascular Ultrasound

Kawasaki Masanori

Additional information is available at the end of the chapter

http://dx.doi.org/10.5772/53955

1. Introduction

In an angioscopic study, Mizuno et al. demonstrated that disruption or erosion of vulnerable plaques and subsequent thromboses are the most frequent cause of acute coronary syndrome (Mizuno et al., 1992). A pathological study by Horie et al. demonstrated that plaque rupture into the lumen of a coronary artery may precede and cause thrombus formation leading to acute myocardial infarction (Horie et al., 1978). The stability of atherosclerotic plaques is related to the histological composition of plaques and the thickness of fibrous caps. Therefore, recognition of the tissue characteristics of coronary plaques is important to understand and prevent acute coronary syndrome. Accurate identification of the tissue characteristics of coronary plaques *in vivo* may allow the identification of vulnerable plaques before the development of acute coronary syndrome.

Recently, intravascular optical coherence tomography (OCT) provides high-resolution, cross-sectional images of tissue in situ and has an axial resolution of 10 μm and a lateral resolution of 20 μm (Tearney et al., 1997; Brezinski et al., 1996). The OCT images of human coronary atherosclerotic plaques obtained in vivo provide additional, more detailed structural information than intravascular ultrasound (IVUS) (Jang et al., 2002; Jang et al., 2005; Kume et al. 2005). Characterizing different types of atherosclerotic plaques on the basis of sensitivity and specificity compared to histological findings to determine plaque vulnerability was established in a previous study (Yabushita et al., 2002). According to this study, the sensitivity and specificity of the classification of the plaque components were sufficient for tissue characterization in clinical settings.

In the 1990's, a new technique was developed that could characterize myocardial tissues by integrated backscatter (IB) analysis of ultrasound images. This technique is capable of providing both conventional two-dimensional echocardiographic images and IB images. Ultrasound backscatter power is proportional to the difference of acoustic characteristic impedance that is determined by the density of tissue multiplied by the speed of sound. In studies of the myocardium, calibrated myocardial IB values were significantly correlated with the relative volume of interstitial fibrosis (Picano, 1990 et al.; Naito et al., 1996). In preliminary studies in vitro, IB values reflected the structural and biochemical composition of atherosclerotic lesion and could differentiate fibrofatty, fatty and calcification of arterial walls (Barziliai et al., 1987; Urbani et al., 1993; Picano et al., 1988). It was also reported that anisotropy of the direction and backscatter power is related to plaque type (De Kroon et al., 1991). Takiuchi et al. found that quantitative tissue characterization using IB ultrasound could identify lipid pool and fibrosis in human carotid and/or femoral arteries (Takiuchi et al., 2000). In the early 2000s, it was reported that IB values measured in vivo in human carotid arteries correlated well with postmortem histological classification (Kawasaki et al., 2001). This new non-invasive technique using IB values could characterize the two-dimensional structures of arterial plaques in vivo. With this technique, plaque tissues were classified based on histopathology into 6 types, i.e. intraplaque hemorrhage, lipid pool, intimal hyperplasia, fibrosis, dense fibrosis, and calcification. This technique was applied in the clinical setting to predict cerebral ischemic lesions after carotid artery stenting. From the analysis of receiver operating characteristic (ROC) curves, a relative intraplaque hemorrhage + lipid pool area of 50% measured by IB ultrasound imaging was the most reliable cutoff value for predicting cerebral ischemic lesions evaluated by diffusion-weighted magnetic resonance imaging after carotid artery stenting (Yamada et al., 2010).

In the next generation, this ultrasound IB technique was applied to coronary arteries by use of intravascular ultrasound (IVUS) (Kawasaki et al., 2010). In the IVUS analysis, 512 vector lines of ultrasound signal around the circumference were analyzed to calculate the IB values. The IB values for each tissue component were calculated using a fast Fourier transform, and expressed as the average power, measured in decibels (dB), of the frequency component of the backscattered signal from a small volume of tissue.

2. Comparison among OCT, IB-IVUS and conventional IVUS for tissue characterization of coronary plaques

Before OCT and IVUS imaging, arteries were warmed to 37 °C in saline. Coronary arteries were imaged with 3.2 F OCT catheters. The position of the interrogating beam on the tissue was monitored by a visible light beam (laser diode, 635 nm) that was coincident with the infrared beam. A total of 128 regions of interest (ROI 0.2 x 0.2 mm) on the OCT images and classified tissue characteristics in the ROIs according to the definitions described in a previous study (Jang et al., 2002). All OCT diagnoses were performed by two skilled readers blinded to the diagnoses based on IVUS and histology. For the comparison with diagnoses based on histology, ROIs from the OCT images in which the diagnoses made by the two OCT readers were identical were used. Conventional IVUS images and IB signals were acquired using an IVUS system (Clear View, Boston Scientific, Natick, Massachusetts) and a 40 MHz intravascular catheter. Definitions of IB values for each histological category were de-

http://dx.doi.org/10.5772/53955

termined by comparing the histological images as reported in a previous study (Kawasaki et al., 2002). To clarify the rotational and cross-sectional position of the included segment, multiple surgical needles were carefully inserted into the coronary arteries before OCT and IVUS imaging to serve as reference points to compare the imaging modalities.

The overall agreement between the OCT and the histological diagnoses was excellent (Cohen's κ = 0.92, 95% CI: 0.85 - 1.00). The overall agreement between the IB-IVUS and histological diagnoses was 0.80 (95% CI: 0.69 - 0.92). The overall agreement of between the conventional IVUS and histological diagnoses was 0.59 (95% CI: 0.42 - 0.77) (Table 1). The overall agreement between the OCT and the IB-IVUS diagnoses was 0.77 (95% CI: 0.65 - 0.90). The overall agreement between the OCT and conventional IVUS diagnoses was 0.62 (95% CI: 0.44 - 0.79) (Table 5). False-positive diagnoses of IB-IVUS and conventional IVUS for lipid pool often contained histological evidence of small amounts of lipid accumulation within a predominantly fibrous lesion. These lesions that included a clinically irrelevant amount of lipid pool were identified as lipid pool by IB-IVUS (n = 3) and echo-lucent by conventional IVUS (n = 5), and reduced the negative predictive values for fibrosis (84% and 74%) (Kawasaki et al., 2006).

	Histology				
	CL	FI	LP	IH	Total
OCT					
Calcification	7	0	0	0	7
Fibrosis	0	86	1	1	88
Lipid pool	0	2	18	0	20
Intimal hyperplasia	0	0	0	6	6
Total	7	88	19	7	121

Cohen's κ = 0.92 (0.85 - 0.99), Weighted κ = 0.92 (0.85 - 1.00)

	Histology				
	CL	FI	LP	IH	Total
IB-IVUS					
Calcification	7	1	0	0	8
Fibrosis	0	77	3	2	82
Lipid pool	0	3	16	0	19
Intimal hyperplasia	0	1	0	4	5
Total	7	82	19	6	114

Cohen's κ = 0.80 (0.69 - 0.92), Weighted κ = 0.79 (0.66 - 0.92)

	Histology				
	CL	FI	LP	IH	Total
Conventional IVUS					
Calcification	7	1	0	0	8
Fibrosis	0	74	5	6	85
Lipid pool	0	5	10	0	15
Intimal hyperplasia	0	0	0	0	0
Total	7	80	15	6	108

Cohen's κ = 0.59 (0.42 - 0.77), Weighted κ = 0.54 (0.35 - 0.72)

CL: calcification, FI: fibrosis, LP: lipid pool, IH: intimal hyperplasia

Table 1. Comparison between imaging diagnosis and histological diagnosis

OCT diagnoses, in which two OCT readers diagnoses were identical, were in excellent agreement with the histological diagnoses. False negative and false positive diagnoses for lipid-rich plaque were seen comparing the OCT images and histological findings (Yabushita et al., 2002). However, false negative diagnoses for lipid-rich plaque, which could be attributed to the limited penetration depth of OCT (1.25 - 2 mm), were not seen because all ROIs were set within the penetration depth of OCT. In addition, false positive diagnoses for lipid-rich plaque, which could be attributed to difficulty of differentiating clinically relevant large lipid pools and insignificant lipid accumulation were not seen because of the small ROIs (0.2 mm x 0.2 mm).

3. Comparison of the thickness of the fibrous cap measured by OCT and IB-IVUS in vivo

During routine selective percutaneous coronary intervention in 42 consecutive patients, a total of 28 cross-sections that consisted of lipid overlaid by a fibrous cap were imaged by both IVUS and optical coherence tomography in 24 patients with stable angina pectoris. A 0.016-inch optical coherence tomography catheter (Imagewire, LightLab Imaging, Inc., Westford, MA) was advanced into the coronary arteries. IB-IVUS and optical coherence tomography (M2 OCT Imaging system, LightLab Imaging, Inc., Westford, MA) were performed in each patient at the same site without significant stenosis as described below.

IB-IVUS images were obtained every one second using an automatic pullback device at a rate of 0.5 mm/sec. optical coherence tomography images were obtained using an automatic pullback system at a rate of 0.5 mm/sec. IB-IVUS images were obtained at 0.5 mm intervals, whereas optical coherence tomography images were obtained at 0.03 mm intervals. Therefore, the segments of coronary artery to compare between the two methods were selected based on the IB-IVUS images. Then, these same coronary segments were identified in optical coherence tomography using the distance from easily-definable side branches and calcification as reference markers to ensure that IB-IVUS and optical coherence tomography were compared at the same site. The cross-sections that did not have sufficient imaging quality to analyze tissue characteristics were excluded from the comparison. In the IB-IVUS analysis, images were processed by a smoothing method that averaged nine IB values in nine pixels located in a square field of the color-coded maps to reduce uneven surfaces of tissue components produced by signal noise.

Fibrous caps that overlaid lipid pool were divided into ROI (every 10° rotation from the center of the vessel lumen) and the average thickness was determined. The average thickness of fibrous cap was determined by averaging the thickness of fibrous cap every 2° within the ROIs (Figure 1). The areas where the radial axis from the center of the vessel lumen crossed the tangential line of the vessel surface with an angle less than a 80° were excluded from the comparison.

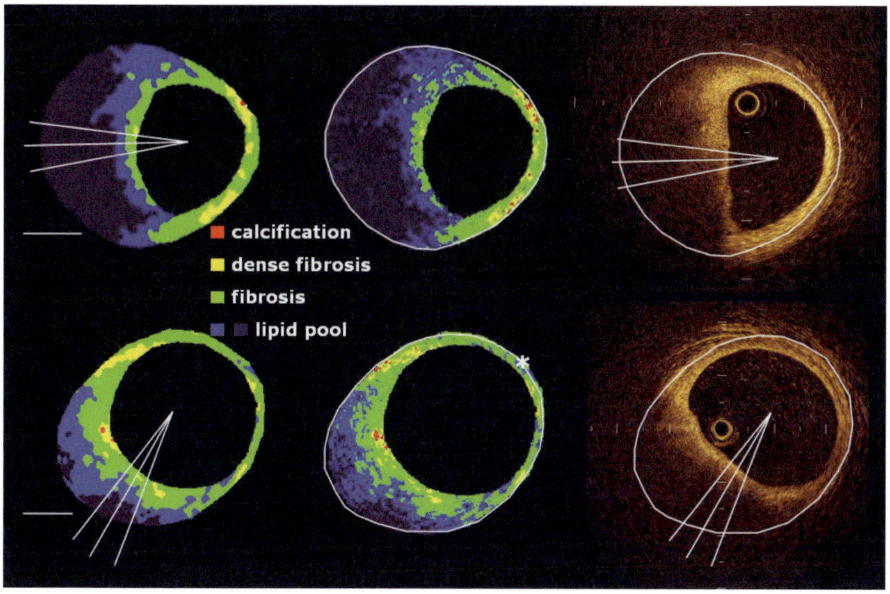

Figure 1. Left) Representative integrated backscatter intravascular ultrasound (IB-IVUS) images processed by a smoothing method. (Middle) Original IB-IVUS images (Right) Corresponding optical coherence tomography. *: attenuation by guide wire. Bar = 1mm.

The thickness of fibrous cap measured by IB-IVUS was significantly correlated with that measured by optical coherence tomography (y = 0.99x – 0.19, r = 0.74, p<0.001) (Figure 2) (Kawasaki et al., 2010).

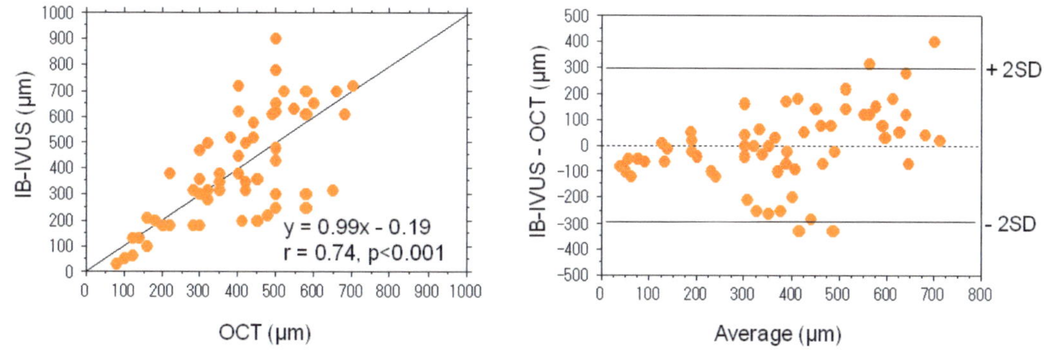

Figure 2. Left: Correlation between the thickness of fibrous cap measured by integrated backscatter intravascular ultrasound and optical coherence tomography. Right: Bland-Altman plot.

A Bland-Altman plot showed that the mean difference between the thickness of fibrous cap measured by IB-IVUS and optical coherence tomography (IB-IVUS - optical coherence tomography) was -2 ± 147 μm (Figure 2). The difference between the two methods appeared to increase as the thickness of the fibrous cap increased (Figure 3).

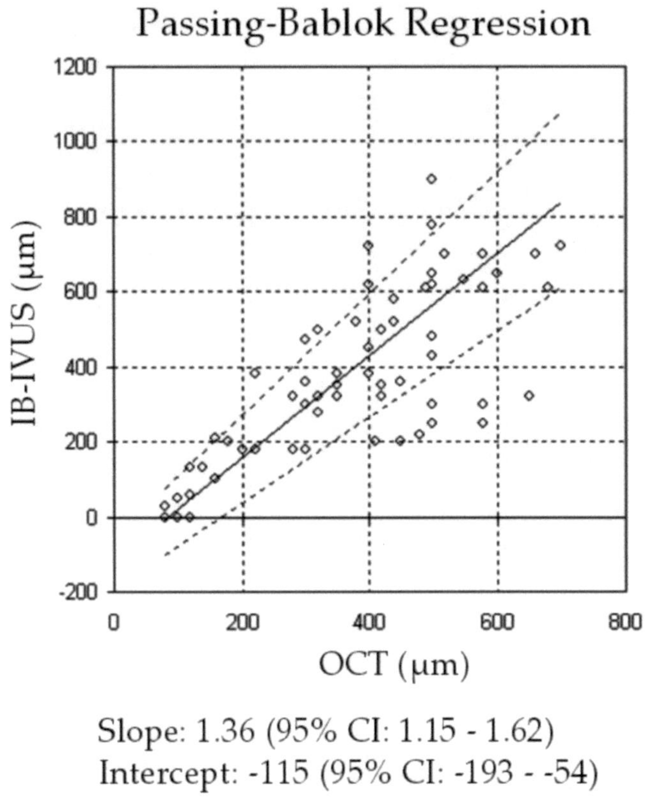

Figure 3. Passing-Bablok regression analysis.

Optical coherence tomography has a better potential for characterizing tissue components located on the near side of the vessel lumen, whereas IB-IVUS has a better potential for characterizing tissue components of entire plaques (Kawasaki et al., 2006).

4. Limitations

There were a few limitations of the ultrasound method. First, the angle-dependence of the ultrasound signal makes tissue characterization unstable when lesions are not perpendicular to the ultrasound axis. Picano et al. reported that angular scattering behavior is large in calcified and fibrous tissues, whereas it is slight to nonexistent in normal and fatty plaques (Picano et al., 1985). According to that report, although there was no crossover of IB values between fibrous and fibrofatty within an angle span of 10°, or between fibrous and fatty within an angle span of 14°, this angle-dependence of the ultrasound signal might be partially responsible for the variation of IB values obtained from each tissue component. There was also a report that demonstrated the degree of angle-dependence of 30 MHz ultrasound in detail (Courtney et al., 2002). In that report, the angle-dependence of 30 MHz ultrasound in the arterial intima and media was 1.11dB/10°. When the 40 MHz catheter was used, the angle dependence increased in arterial tissue. This angle-dependence of the ultrasound signal may decrease the diagnostic accuracy for differentiating tissue components.

Second, the guidewire was not used in the process of imaging because the present studies were performed *ex vivo*. Imaging artifacts *in vivo* due to the guidewire may decrease the diagnostic accuracy. However, removal of the guidewire during imaging after completing the intervention procedure and/or excluding the area behind calcification from the analysis may be necessary in the clinical setting to eliminate this problem. Finally, detecting thrombus from a single IVUS cross-section was not possible because we usually look at multiple IVUS images over time for speckling, scintillation, motion and blood flow in the "microchannel" (Mintz et al., 2001). The analysis of IB values in multiple cross-sections over time is required for the detection of thrombus.

Author details

Kawasaki Masanori

Address all correspondence to: masanori@ya2.so-net.ne.jp

Department of Cardiology, Gifu University Graduate School of Medicine, Japan

References

[1] Barziliai B, Shffitz JE, Miller JG, Sobel BE. (1987). Quantitative ultrasonic characterization of the nature of atherosclerotic plaques in human aorta. Circ Res.Vol 60: 459-63.

[2] Brezinski ME, Tearney GJ, Bouma BE, Izatt JA, Hee MR, Swanson EA, Southern JF, Fujimoto JG. (1996). Optical coherence tomography for optical biopsy: properties and demonstration of vascular pathology. Circulation Vol 93:1206–1213.

[3] Brezinski ME, Tearney GJ, Weissman NJ, Boppart SA, Bouma BE, Hee MR, Weyman AE, Swanson EA, Southern JF, Fujimoto JG. (1997). Assessing atherosclerotic plaque morphology: comparison of optical coherence tomography and high frequency intravascular ultrasound. Heart Vol 77:397-403.

[4] Brown BG, Zhao XQ, Sacco DE, Albers JJ. (1993). Lipid lowering and plaque regression. New insights into prevention of plaque disruption and clinical events in coronary disease. Circulation. Vol 87:1781-91.

[5] Courtney BK, Robertson AL, Maehara A, Luna J, Kitamura K, Morino Y, et al. (2002). Effect of transducer position on backscattered intensity in coronary arteries. Ultrasound in Med & Biol. Vol 28:81-91.

[6] De Kroon MGM, van der Wal LF, Gussenhoven WJ, Rijsterborgh H, Bom N. (1991). Backscatter directivity and integrated backscatter power of arterial tissue. Int J Card Imaging.Vol 6:265-75.

[7] Horie, T., Sekiguchi, M., Hirosawa, K. (1978). Coronary thrombosis in pathogenesis of acute myocardial infarction. Histopathological study of coronary arteries in 108 necropsied cases using serial section. Br Heart J Vol. 40:153-61.

[8] Jang IK, Bouma BE, Kang DH, Park SJ, Park SW, Seung KB, Choi KB, Shishkov M, Schlendorf K, Pomerantsev E, Houser SL, Aretz HT, Tearney GJ. (2002). Visualization of coronary atherosclerotic plaques in patients using optical coherence tomography: comparison with intravascular ultrasound. J Am Coll Cardiol Vol 39:604–609.

[9] Jang IK, Tearney GJ, MacNeill B, Takano M, Moselewski F, Iftima N, Shishkov M, Houser S, Aretz HT, Halpern EF, Bouma BE. (2005). In vivo characterization of coronary atherosclerotic plaque by use of optical coherence tomography. Circulation Vol 111:1551-1555.

[10] Kawasaki M, Takatsu H, Noda T, Ito Y, Kunishima A, Arai M, Nishigaki K, Takemura G, Morita N, Minatoguchi S, Fujiwara H. (2001). Non-invasive tissue characterization of human atherosclerotic lesions in carotid and femoral arteries by ultrasound integrated backscatter. -Comparison between histology and integrated backscatter images before and after death- J Am Coll Cardiol. Vol 38:486-92

[11] Kawasaki M, Takatsu H, Noda T, Sano K, Ito Y, Hayakawa K, Tsuchiya K, Arai M, Nishigaki K, Takemura G, Minatoguchi S, Fujiwara T, Fujiwara H. (2002) In vivo quantitative tissue characterization of human coronary arterial plaques by use of integrated backscatter intravascular ultrasound and comparison with angioscopic findings. Circulation Vol 105:2487-2492.

[12] Kawasaki M, Bouma BE, Bressner J, Houser SL, Nadkarni SK, MacNeill BD, Jang IK, Fujiwara H, Tearney GJ. (2006). Diagnostic accuracy of optical coherence tomography and integrated backscatter intravascular ultrasound images for tissue characterization of human coronary plaques. J Am Coll Cardiol Vol 48:81-8.

[13] Kawasaki M, Hattori A, Ishihara Y, Okubo M, Nishigaki K, Takemura G, Saio M, Takami T, Minatoguchi S. (2010). Tissue characterization of coronary plaques and assessment of thickness of fibrous cap using integrated backscatter intravascular ultrasound. Comparison with histology and optical coherence tomography. Circ J Vol 74:2641-48.

[14] Kume T, Akasaka T, Kawamoto T, Watanabe N, Toyota E, Neishi Y, Sukmawan R, Sadahira Y, Yoshida K. (2005). Assessment of coronary intima-media thickness by optical coherence tomography: comparison with intravascular ultrasound. Circ J Vol 69:903-907.

[15] Mintz GS, Nissen SE, Anderson WD, Bailey SR, Erbel R, Fitzgerald PJ, Pinto FJ, Rosenfield K, Siegel RJ, Tuzcu EM, Yock PG. (2001). American College of Cardiology

clinical expert consensus document on standards for acquisition, measurement and reporting of intravascular ultrasound studies (IVUS). A report of the American College of Cardiology task force on clinical expert consensus documents developed in collaboration with the European society of cardiology endorsed by the society of cardiac angiography and interventions. J Am Coll Cardiol. Vol 37:1478-92.

[16] Mizuno K, Satomura K, Miyamoto A, Arakawa K, Shibuya T, Arai T, Kurita A, Nakamura H, Ambrose JA. (1992). Angioscopic evaluation of coronary artery thrombi in acute coronary syndromes. N Engl J Med Vol 326:287-91.

[17] Naito J, Masuyama T, Mano T, Kondo H, Yamamoto K, Nagano R, Doi Y, Hori M, Kamada T. (1996). Ultrasound myocardial tissue characterization in the patients with dilated cardiomyopathy: Value in noninvasive assessment of myocardial fibrosis. Am Heart J. Vol 131:115-21.

[18] Picano E, Landini L, Distante A, Salvadori M, Lattanzi F, Masini M, L'Abbate A. (1985). Angle dependence of ultrasonic backscatter in arterial tissues: a study in vitro. Circulation.Vol 72:572-6.

[19] Picano E, Landini L, Lattanzi F, Salvadori M, Benassi A, L'Abbate A. (1988). Time domain echo pattern evaluation from normal and atherosclerotic arterial walls: a study in vitro. Circulation. Vol 77:654-9.

[20] Picano E, Pelosi G, Marzilli M, Lattanzi F, Benassi A, Landini L, L'Abbate A. (1990). In vivo quantitative ultrasonic evaluation of myocardial fibrosis in humans. Circulation. Vol 81:58-64.

[21] Takiuchi S, Rakugi H, Honda K, Masuyama T, Hirata N, Ito H, Sugimoto K, Yanagitani Y, Moriguchi K, Okamura A, Higaki J, Ogihara T. (2000). Quantitative ultrasonic tissue characterization can identify high-risk atherosclerotic alteration in human carotid arteries. Circulation Vol 102:766-70.

[22] Tearney GJ, Brezinski ME, Bouma BE, Boppart SA, Pitris C, Southern JF, Fujimoto JG. (1997). In vivo endoscopic optical biopsy with optical coherence tomography. Science Vol 276:2037–2039.

[23] Urbani MP, Picano E, Parenti G, Mazzarisi A, Fiori L, Paterni M, Pelosi G, Landini L. (1993). In vivo radiofrequency-based ultrasonic tissue characterization of the atherosclerotic plaque. Stroke. Vol 24:1507-12.

[24] Yabushita H, Bouma BE, Houser SL, Aretz HT, Jang IK, Schlendorf KH, Kauffman CR, Shishkov M, Kang DH, Halpern EF, Tearney GJ. (2002). Characterization of human atherosclerosis by optical coherence tomography. Circulation 106:1640-1645.

[25] Yamada K, Kawasaki M, Yoshimura S, Enomoto Y, Asano T, Minatoguchi S, Iwama T. (2010). Prediction of silent ischemic lesions after carotid artery stenting using integrated backscatter ultrasound and magnetic resonance imaging. Atherosclerosis Vol 208:161-6.

Section 3

Engineering

Chapter 8

Full Field Optical Coherence Microscopy: Imaging and Image Processing for Micro-Material Research Applications

Bettina Heise, Stefan Schausberger and
David Stifter

Additional information is available at the end of the chapter

http://dx.doi.org/10.5772/53509

1. Introduction

Non-destructive optical imaging and probing techniques have found entrance and success in material sciences favoured by their non-invasive investigation character. X-ray computer tomography (CT) applied in a different size scale (e.g. as micro-CT and nano-CT [1]) is well established as a non-destructive technique in the field of material inspection. CT imaging delivers highly contrasted images of the internal of the specimens. It includes information about inclusions or cavities, and about the size and distribution of particles and pores within the technical material. Furthermore, ultrasound and acousto-optic imaging may also provide valuable insights into internal cracks and flaws, density or concentration variations, or even features as material elasticity. Although both techniques are versatile for use in different applications in material analysis, they also show restrictions: for biological samples in particular, there are the hazards of X-ray radiation; the techniques obey typical resolution limits in relation to the sample dimensions, or they require an additional coupling medium as in ultrasonic imaging (US).

With the availability of powerful broadband near infrared wavelength (NIR) light sources some decades ago, low-coherence interferometry (LCI) for the investigation of scattering or semi-transparent materials has become an alternative to CT and US methods. In 1991, optical coherence tomography (OCT) was introduced as an imaging technique by [2]. At the beginning, OCT mainly gained ground in the field of medical diagnostics, in particular in ophthalmology, representing a novel visualization technique for different ocular diseases, followed by numerous applications in cardiology, dentistry, dermatology, nephrology, amongst others

[3-6]. The imaging capabilities of OCT for subcutaneous assessment of the specimen need particular mention, and in the case of OCT being realized endoscopically [7], OCT can deliver valuable tissue information from various internal positions and sites within the human body.

The capability and specific use of OCT for non-medical purposes as in material sciences or arts has been recognized relatively late, arising with metrology and topographic profiling of microelectronic circuits [8] and optical components (which rather resembles optical time domain reflectometry (ODTR) or white light profilometry). The optical inspection of glass fibers and ceramic parts need to be mentioned, as well as further applications in art conservation (providing information about the conservation state of paintings [9] or about cracks and defects in porcelain and jade stones [10]), in paper inspection [11], or in dynamic process monitoring [12]. Recently, the use of OCT technique for the characterization of internal structures in polymer and compound materials such as multilayer foils, fiber-epoxy composites, or different types of extruded plastics and foams have become a research focus in polymer sciences [13].

Intensity-based OCT provides structural information about the probed specimen. The conventional modality can be modified by different polarization- or phase-sensitive functional extensions (naming e.g. polarization-sensitive OCT (PS-OCT), differential phase contrast OCT (DPC-OCT), or Doppler OCT), where also birefringence, phase or frequency can be extracted locally and in a depth–resolved way. Thereby additionally information about the specimen's functional behaviour (as optical anisotropies, elasticity, internal strain-stress distributions, or internal flow fields) can be gained [14, 15].

Recently reported OCT trends focus on various aspects. These trends are governed by the aim:

- to speed up the image acquisition time by ultra-fast scanning setups, working in Fourier domain and using special swept laser sources [16],
- to miniaturize the setup by using integrated optical techniques [17],
- to apply multi-modal imaging techniques and combining OCT with other imaging methods like fluorescence microscopy and spectroscopy [18] or hyper-spectral imaging techniques [19],
- to exploit non-linear effects in the signal like second harmonic generation or multi-photon imaging [20, 21],
- to work under a full-field imaging regime (instead of raster scanning techniques, as is typical for conventional OCT imaging) and in combination with microscopic elements to lead to so-called full-field optical coherence microscopy (FF-OCM) or full field OCT (FF-OCT) [22],
- to be supplemented by sophisticated image processing [23] or data analysis on graphics processing units (GPU) [24].

In this book chapter, we discuss the last two points in particular: First, full-field optical coherent microscopy -- its physical principles, similarities and differences to comparable OCT applications, its use for material characterization and dynamical inspections, and possible contrast modifications. Secondly, we discuss the enrichment of FF-OCM imaging by some illustrative

http://dx.doi.org/10.5772/53509

examples for image processing, showing the potential given by different mathematical algorithms in the field of object analysis.

2. FF-OCM imaging techniques

2.1. Physical principle

OCT and OCM imaging techniques are based on the principle of low-coherence interferometry. Both methods exploit the (low) coherence properties of broadband light sources, allowing for tuneable depth positioning of the narrow coherence gate/range within the sample. But whereas OCT (working in time- or frequency domain) represents a raster scanning technique probing along the beam line and sensing the reflected light point by point, FF-OCM produces interferometric images parallel to the sample surface. The entire field of view at the sample is illuminated at once by a low-coherent light beam, and the reflected light from an extended lateral region is received by a CCD or CMOS camera as detectors.

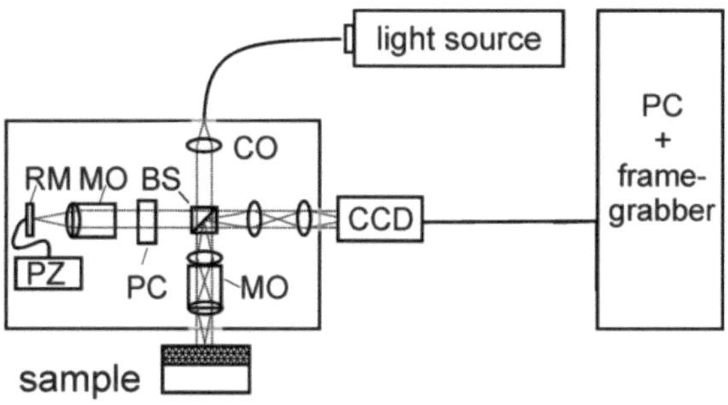

Figure 1. Scheme of the optical setup of the (time domain) FF-OCM realized in a Michelson/Linnik interferometer configuration, (BS: beamsplitter, CO: collimator, PC: path compensation, MO: microscopic objectives, RM: reference mirror, PZ: piezo translator).

In general, a FF-OCM setup is established in a Michelson/Linnik interferometric configuration (or for special purposes in some modifications as in Mach-Zehnder configuration), as depicted in Figure 1, with two identical optical elements assemblies (i.e. using the same micro-objectives and dispersion compensations) for both the sample and the reference arm. Applying broadband light sources for illumination and guaranteeing a homogeneously illuminated area, the incoming wave field is divided into sample and reference wave field. Both wave fields are reflected either by the sample or the reference mirror and superposed at the detector.

Interference can only occur when the optical path length of sample and reference arm are nearly identical with respect to the coherence length of the source. Then interferometric fringe images can be recorded within the coherence gate whose width is determined by the (temporal) coherence length of the source. The ratio of optical path length of sample to reference arm may be continuously changed by altering the position of the sample mounted at an axial motorized translation stage. The reference mirror is placed on an oscillating piezoelectric translation stage (PZT). The PZT is driven either by a sinusoidal or by a saw tooth periodic oscillation. By displacing the reference mirror, a shift of the optical path length in fractions of the wavelength is introduced in a discrete or continuous way. It allows the recording of several phase shifted interferometric fringe images. By mathematical combination of the mutual phase-shifted images the FF-OCM reflectivity image can be obtained by a subsequent demodulation.

2.2. Light sources and resolution aspects

The choice of light source is of crucial importance for the penetration depth and the resolution achieved. It should be considered with respect to the planned application.

Similar to OCT, the axial resolution in FF-OCM is determined by the temporal coherence length of the source, which is proportional to the ratio $\lambda^2/\Delta\lambda$, with the wavelength λ and the spectral width $\Delta\lambda$ of the applied light source. The lateral resolution is mainly characterized by the numerical aperture (NA) of the objectives similar to conventional microscopy: high NA objectives increase lateral resolution. But high NA may also become dominant for axial resolution in FF-OCM [25], as the depth of field becomes very narrow for higher NA objectives. By careful dynamic focusing coherence gate and focus position of objectives can be matched within the investigated material.

As the penetration depth increases with the wavelength λ, light sources in the NIR range with a central wavelength of 1000 -- 1500 nm are often to be preferred to light sources at 800 nm, particularly for imaging technical structures, where water absorption does not play any role. However, axial resolution is reduced with increasing wavelength. Furthermore, the camera detection system also has to be adapted to the requested wavelength range using InGaAs-based detector types, which may cause higher financial costs.

For the light source itself, super-luminescence diodes [26], femto-second (fs) pulse laser [27], diode laser pumped super-continuum sources [28, 29], or thermal light sources [30] have been described in different illumination concepts, each with their advantages and drawbacks. Thermal light sources best prevent speckle noise and are not hampered by side-lobes as in the case of fs-laser or SLD. However, the adjustment of the setup is challenging. Halogen flash light sources are used for stroboscopic imaging and obtain an axial resolution less than 1 µm. A sophisticatedly tuned image acquisition scheme is required therefore. Broadband fs-pulse lasers with high repetition rates in the range of hundred MHz are another alternative for high resolution imaging; however these lasers are expensive. The use of nano-second pulse lasers is suggested in [31] as a valuable compromise: they achieve reasonable repetition rates while reducing costs.

In summary, the factors of resolution, penetration and costs must be weighed against each other when determining which light source to use in investigating technical materials or biological samples.

3. Demodulation

In interferometric imaging, an interference fringe pattern $I(x,y)$ can be described as

$$I(x,y) = B(x,y) + A(x,y)\cos(\phi(x,y)), \tag{1}$$

where $A(x,y)$ represents the amplitude modulation, $\varphi(x,y)$ the phase modulation, and $B(x,y)$ is determined by any background illumination or surface characteristics.

Introducing multiple phase shifts $\varphi_n(x,y)$ between the different frames, a sequence $I_n(x,y)$ of interferometric images at a fixed depth position z may be described as

$$I_n(x,y) = B(x,y) + A(x,y)\cos(\phi(x,y) + \Delta\phi_n). \tag{2}$$

The aim of demodulation is to decode the amplitude (or phase) modulation, thereby extracting the interference fringe envelope at each lateral position. The amplitude modulation $A(x,y)$ is characterized by the local reflectivity of the sample at each depth position z (similar to OCT), and so the reflectivity map can be obtained by amplitude demodulation. It should be mentioned here that the phase/frequency modulation $\varphi(x,y)$ of the fringe pattern can also be exploited. It reveals details about local deformations of structures in the sub-wavelength range or about minimal refractive index changes in the imaged sample. However, reliable phase information can only be extracted from regions where sufficient amplitude modulation is guaranteed.

Different phase stepping approaches are used for data acquisition and demodulation. Generally, a set of phase-shifted interferometric fringe images (usually 4---8 frames) are recorded at each axial position of the sample. Assuming an equidistant sampling over the mirror oscillation, the amplitude and phase map can be obtained by a complex addition of the shifted interference fringes, taking into account the phase shifts $\Delta\varphi_n(x,y)$

$$A(x,y) = abs\left(\sum_{n=1}^{N} I_n(x,y)\exp[i\Delta\phi_n(x,y)\right) \tag{3}$$

and

$$\phi(x,y) = \arg\left(\sum_{n=1}^{N} I_n(x,y)\exp[i\Delta\phi_n(x,y)\right). \tag{4}$$

Different approaches towards the appropriate number of phase steps or towards the influence of non-equally spaced phase shifts on the demodulation accuracy are reported in literature [32].

For four shifted images with phase distances of $\pi/2$ the demodulation equations are simplified to simple trigonometric relations, for higher frame numbers averaging effects can be exploited for accuracy. Nevertheless, it should be mentioned that for monitoring dynamic processes, the ideal is to reduce the frame number to one frame (or in practise to two frames). With a dual shot imaging setup, two π–shifted frames can be obtained in a sequential way, whereas in single shot configurations a two channel pathway is assembled, exploiting polarization or diffraction effects, and a phase shift of π between the two spatially separated frames is introduced.

By building the difference image between the two frames the background term $B(x,y)$ can be reduced. This background-free difference image can now be demodulated with respect to amplitude or phase by so-called single frame processing methods [33].

These methods are based on analytic signal theory. In particular, the 2D analytic approach [34] and the monogenic approach [35] should be mentioned for single frame demodulation. In the 2D analytic approach amplitude and phase map can be expressed as

$$A(x,y)=\sqrt{f^2(x,y)+{H_x}^2 f(x,y)+{H_y}^2 f(x,y)+{H_T}^2 f(x,y)} \tag{5}$$

$$\phi(x,y)=\operatorname{atan}\left(\frac{\sqrt{{H_x}^2 f(x,y)+{H_y}^2 f(x,y)+{H_T}^2 f(x,y)}}{f(x,y)}\right), \tag{6}$$

where H_x, H_y, and H_T represent the partial and total Hilbert transform [36] applied to the difference image $f(x,y)$.

A two frame demodulation scheme is based on the monogenic signal approach [37, 38] with amplitude and phase map expressed as

$$A(x,y)=\sqrt{f^2(x,y)+{R_x}^2 f(x,y)+{R_y}^2 f(x,y)} \tag{7}$$

$$\phi(x,y)=\operatorname{atan}\left(\frac{\sqrt{{R_x}^2 f(x,y)+{R_y}^2 f(x,y)}}{f(x,y)}\right), \tag{8}$$

where R_x and R_y represent the two components of the Riesz transform given as

$$R_x=\frac{x}{2\pi r^3}\otimes(.)=\frac{\cos\vartheta}{2\pi r^2}\otimes(.) \quad \text{and} \quad R_y=\frac{y}{2\pi r^3}\otimes(.)=\frac{\sin\vartheta}{2\pi r^2}\otimes(.),$$

where $\otimes$ (.) denotes the convolution applied on the image $f(x,y)$, and (r, ϑ) the polar coordinates of radius and angle. Furthermore, by the ratio of both Riesz components the orientation of fringes or structures can be determined. This approach is to be preferred in case of aiming at a more isotropic response of the demodulation scheme, as briefly illustrated in Figure 2.

The development of these single shot methods is an on-going process, especially in the case of exploiting the potential of FF-OCM for dynamic scenes. Alternative approaches use micro-mirror devices [39] instead of conventional optical components, such as a Wollaston prism for a partial beam shifting [40].

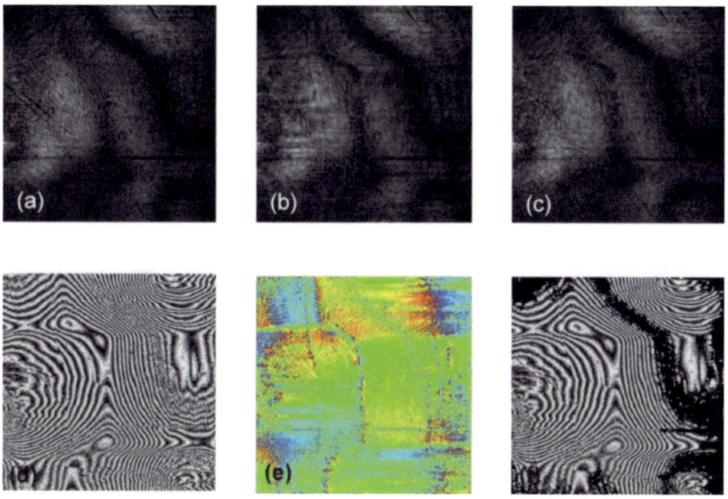

Figure 2. Comparison of demodulation schemes: (a-c) demodulated amplitude map applying (a) phase stepping, (b) 2D analytic signal approach, (c) monogenic signal approach as demodulation methods, (d) and (e) phase and fringe orientation map applying the monogenic approach, and (f) phase map with a superimposed reliability mask (based on the amplitude map for confidence estimation). The good match between the phase stepping approach (a) (assumed as ground truth) and the both single frame approaches (b) and (c) can be seen.

4. FF-OCM for technical material imaging

In the last decade, OCT imaging has been established as non-destructive method for investigating technical structures and processes. It partly benefited from the continuous improvement and perfection of OCT technique in numerous applications in the field of medicine. This newly gained knowledge was also transferred into the field of material research. In particular, functional OCT extension techniques such as PS-OCT, DPC-OCT, elastography-OCT [41, 42], or Doppler OCT have been introduced into the evaluation of technical sample structures and related material properties and features.

In the field of FF-OCM, a similar development from medical and biological applications to technical applications can also be observed. Typical samples, which may be probed by FF-OCM, are found in polymer materials as multilayer or filler enriched polymer foils, where the subsequent layers and filler particles can be visualized, (Figure 3a, b); fiber-reinforced materials of different type of manufacturing, (Figure 3c, d), or semi-transparent minerals, (Figure 3e, f). The quality assessment of organic coatings for a consistent material protection should be named as a further interesting application field of FF-OCM.

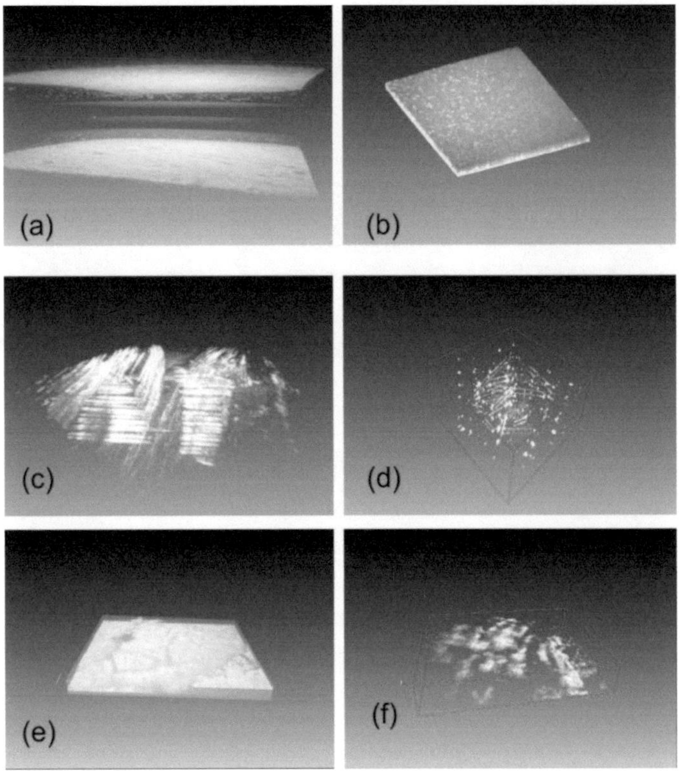

Figure 3. Examples of technical specimens investigated by FF-OCM: 3D volume rendering of a (a) multilayer foil and (b) functional polymer foil containing metallic micro-particles, (c) and (d) inside of a fiber-reinforced polymer sample with casted woven fibers in epoxy-resin (c) and with extruded short glass fibers in polypropylene (d) as filler materials, (e) Halit mineral specimen (finding place: Bolivia) with (f) included defect structures. The imaging volume yields depending on the sample ~ 1x1x0.2...0.4 mm^3.

In the next section, we consider in detail the abilities of FF-OCM to explore fiber-reinforced polymers or polymer materials under stress, which often have been imaged also by conventional OCT. We further consider the potential of different polarization sensitive OCT and OCM versions.

4.1. FF-OCM for characterization of fiber–reinforced polymers

Fiber reinforced polymers play an important role in the design of novel materials with specific and tuneable properties. The characterization of the internal fiber distributions within the matrix material can provide insights into material features or highlight potentials for improving the manufacturing process. Fiber structures differ with respect to their fiber concentration, with respect to the different manufacturing conditions (e.g. woven or randomly aligned fibers), or with respect to their functional role as filler components in materials.

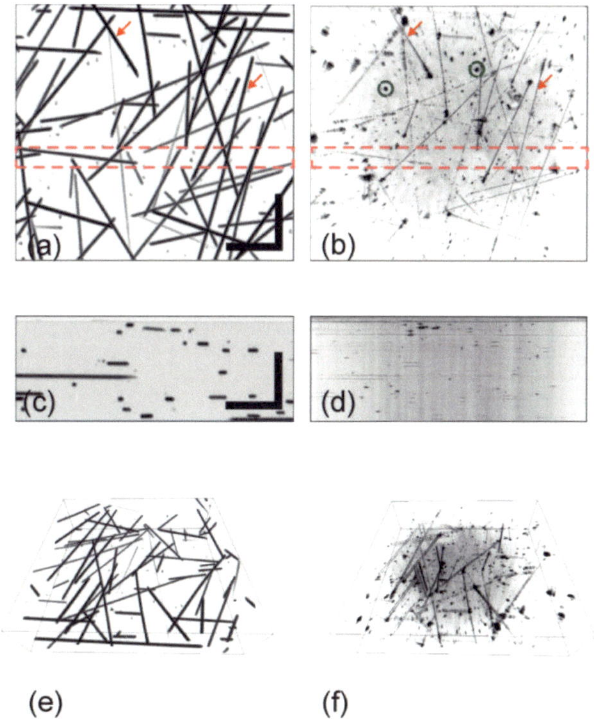

Figure 4. Comparison of the visualization characteristics between micro-CT and FF-OCM: Corresponding sites of the SGF-PP sample probed by micro-CT (left) and by FF-OCM (right), depicted as horizontal (top), cross-sectional (middle) and 3D view (bottom). Reprinted from [31], with permission from Elsevier, © 2012.

Often micro-CT is the method of choice for analyzing these polymer samples. In [31] polymer sheets of polypropylene (PP) containing short glass-fiber (SGF) as fillers are investigated applying both techniques, CT and FF-OCM, to compare and add their partly complementary imaging abilities for the visualization of inclusions or defects. Figure 4 shows a 3D image stack of a SGF-PP composite recorded with either technique. Note the good match between both techniques with respect to fiber localization and detection. Furthermore, complimentary information can be extracted through CT and OCM: the total volume of the fiber is visible in the CT reconstruction; in FF-OCM reconstruction, the reflection signal at front- and backside of the fibers are visible, and we can recognize various crystallization artefacts and micro-cracks there. Due to the low X-ray absorption difference these artefacts are not visible in CT imaging.

After probing, the recorded data can be improved by image processing. Mathematical image enhancement, for example, allows to reduce noise and illumination effects or to adjust the contrast [43]. The application of a background correction based on a morphological filtering for the SGF-PP sample is illustrated in Figure 5.

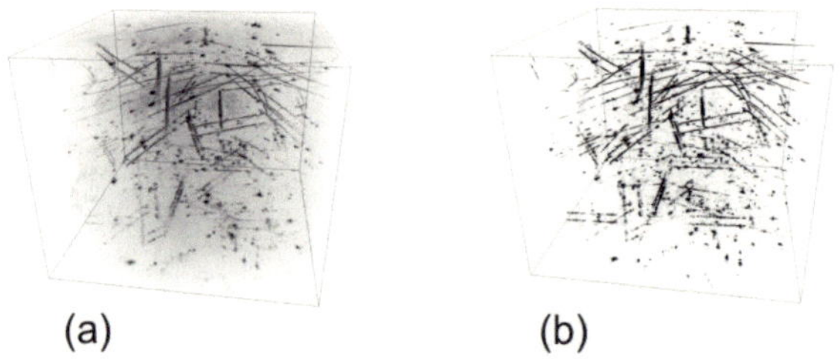

Figure 5. volume rendering of a SGF-PP compound: (a) original FF-OCM image stack, (b) enhanced structures after morphological background correction and noise filtering. The imaging volume yields ~ 1x1x0.3 mm^3. Reprinted from [31], with permission from Elsevier, © 2012.

A subsequent wavelet and shearlet based filtering and optimization approach [44] can separate the detected and pre-processed structures (Figure 6a) into fibers and spherical artefacts or cracks. This is done in a mathematical way, (Figure 6b and c).

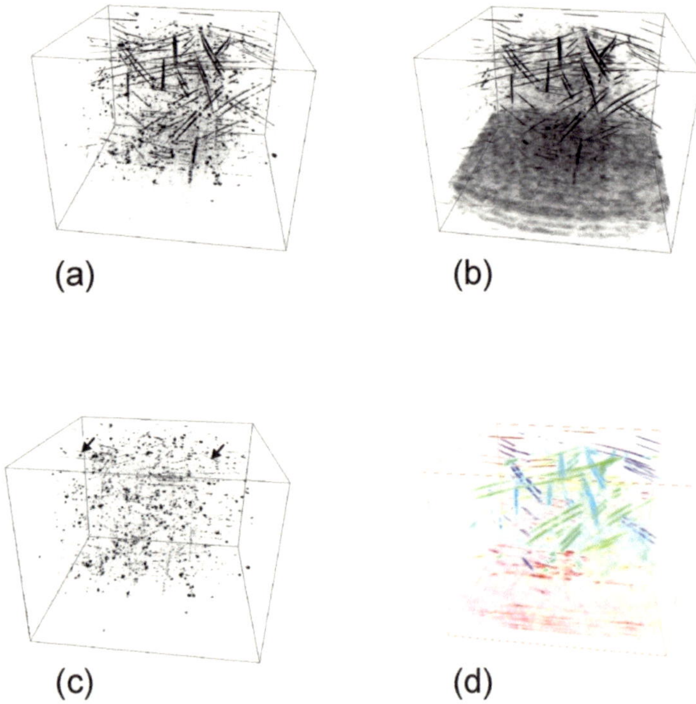

Figure 6. Illustration of the object separation, based mathematically on a shearlet and wavelet approach: the complete pre-processed 3D image stack (SFGF-PP sample) (a) and mathematically separated 3D stacks, containing fibers (b) and crystallization defects (c) as components. The local orientation of fibers (d), extracted by a monogenic signal approach, is represented in a colour encoded version. Reprinted from: [31], with permission from Elsevier, © 2012.

Finally, we can determine the local orientation of the fibers by means of a monogenic (complex-valued) signal approach, as can be seen in Figure 6d. For the orientation estimation, the MonogenicJ toolbox of EPFL has been used [45].

4.2. FF-OCM for monitoring strained /stressed polymers

The previous fiber-composite application is related to a static imaging and analysis of the polymer sample. Now we discuss the ability of FF-OCM to monitor dynamic scenes, e.g. polymers under load in a tensile testing. In [46] we have already reported a similar example: There, a rubber particle filled PP polymer under load was investigated in a tensile testing unit by spectral domain OCT. A local polymer region showing necking and flowing behaviour versus a static region could be distinguished after reaching the yield point. By calculating the speckle variance map over a temporal sequence of OCT reflectivity images, the static and dynamic region could be visually enhanced and the front of material flow could be identified (Figure 7).

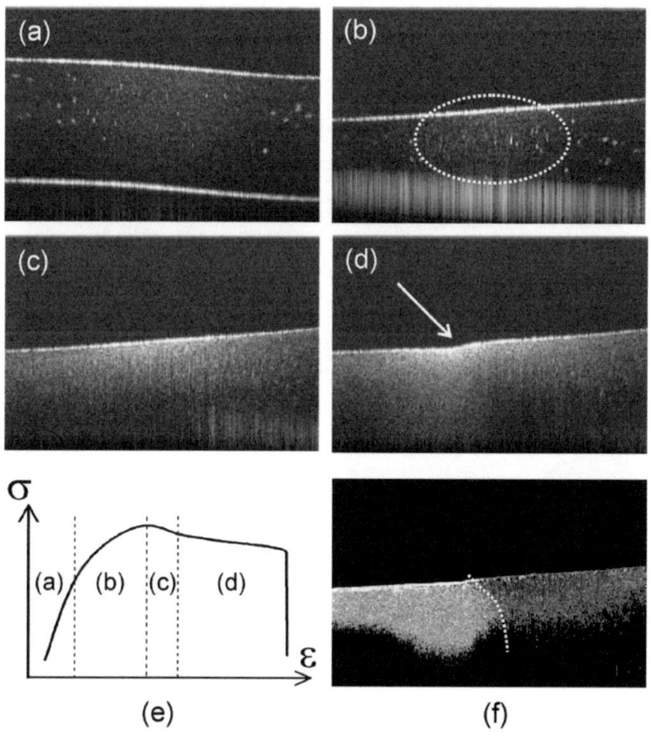

Figure 7. Dynamic stretching process monitored by SD-OCT: (a)-(d) single-frame reflectivity scans (cross sectional views) by OCT imaging showing a rubber particle filled PP polymer test bar (thickness: 1mm) under increasing tensile load, observed at different times. (e) Simultaneously measured strain-stress curve, indicating different regions which correspond to the sample stages (a)-(d): (a) linear elastic region, (b) non-linear elastic region and beginning of plastic deformation leading to increased scattering, (c) permanent plastic deformation after crossing the yield point and on-set of necking, (d) pronounced necking (necking front indicated with arrow), finally leading to fracture. (f) Statistical evaluation (speckle variance map) of cross-sections taken between regimes (c) and (d) to visualize front of material flow during necking, as indicated by dotted line. Reprinted from [46], with permission from OSA, ©2010.

A similar experiment was repeated during FF-OCM measurements [47]. A tensile test unit was included in the sample arm of the interferometric FF-OCM setup, and the focus of the imaging was fixed at a defined depth position of interest. Again, the sample consists of a thin SGF-PP polymer sheet. We could also verify a (horizontal) flowing behaviour of the polymer matrix along the extending fracture in the material by the FF-OCM imaging technique as well. In addition, the normalized variance (second moment) and skewness (third moment) maps are computed over a temporal sequence of reflectivity images, (Figure 8). Furthermore, we also monitored the jumping up and final breaking of fibers within the polymer.

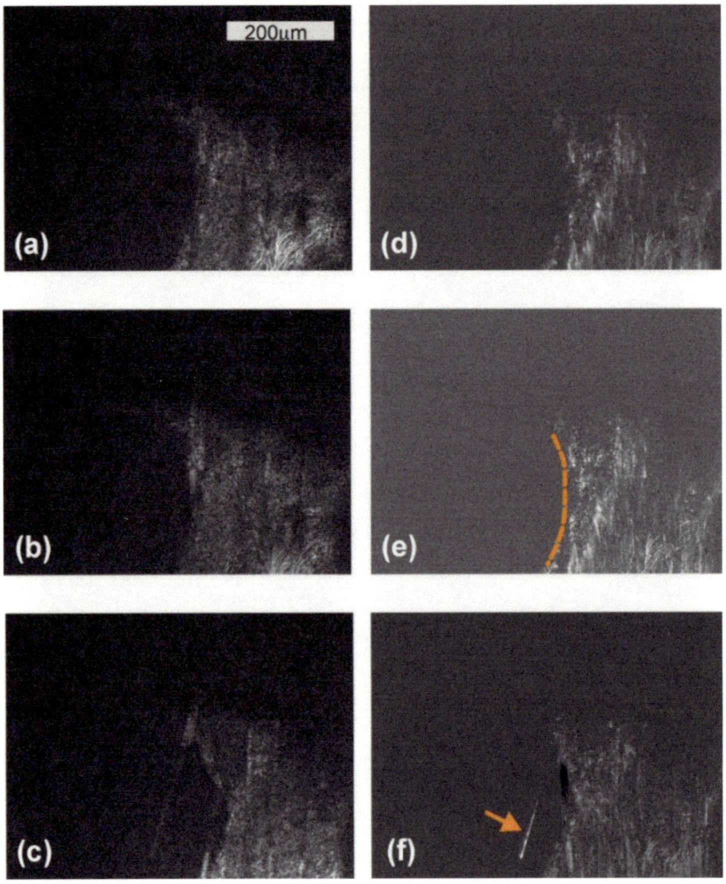

Figure 8. Dynamic tensile test imaging: (a)-(c): single-frame reflectivity scans (horizontal en-face views) by FF-OCM imaging, showing a glass fiber-reinforced polymer test sample under increasing tensile load, observed at different times. Statistical evaluation: (d) normalized variance map, (e) and (f) skewness map at the beginning and at a later point in time (computed over a temporal sequence of reflectivity scans). The front of material flow/fracture line is indicated by the dashed line, the arrow indicates a fiber leaping up.

To visualize dynamic processes without motion artefacts, a sufficient frame rate is required which matches the process dynamics. To guarantee high speed imaging in FF-OCM, on the one hand a suitable demodulation approach (see Section 3) has to be applied, and on the other hand a fast enough detection system has to be chosen. Alternatively to the CCD camera used in static FF-OCM imaging applications, we recently applied a scientific CMOS (sCMOS) camera [47] for dynamic imaging. This enables us to obtain a frame rate that is sufficiently fast compared to CCD, that still has an acceptable sensitivity (70 dB with 4 x 4 binning) and is combined with an almost linear response over the 16-bit imaging range.

4.3. PS-FF-OCM imaging

Polarization sensitive (PS) versions of OCT allow us to obtain functional information from the material: its optical anisotropies and birefringence properties. As in the case of polymers, conclusions can be drawn about internal stress or strain fields in the PS probed sample: The strain fields can be explained e.g. by stress induced during the solidification or extrusion process. A reorientation of polymer molecular chains to a preferred linear alignment under stretching conditions or an already inherent orientational birefringence may cause the optically anisotropic behaviour of polymer material. The temporal evolution of such stress states caused by dynamic processes such as loading, stretching, extrusion, crystallization, or heating can be suitably monitored by PS-OCT.

A PS-OCT imaging can be accomplished by extending a conventional OCT setup with additional polarization optical components (i.e. polarizer, wave plates, and polarizing beam splitters) as illustrated schematically in Figure 9. Dual channel detection with respect to both orthogonal polarization directions can now be performed. In addition to the intensity-based reflectivity, further phase retardation and optical axis orientation can be determined. Using Stokes vector formalism, also the degree of polarization uniformity (DOPU) or birefringence (as change of retardation over depth) can be examined [48].

Conventional FF-OCM may be extended as well to a polarization sensitive FF-OCM version (PS-FF-OCM) [49]. The extension is realized similar to the time domain PS-OCT configuration described above. Here, either two cameras are applied using a conventional polarizing beamsplitter, or the images are taken by a single camera with a Wollaston prism mounted at the front. The Wollaston prism splits the two orthogonally polarized image components which are recorded at a single CCD area detector. It should be mentioned that a very good adjustment of the camera system or a pixel-to-pixel registration between the two image components is necessary to reduce artefacts of slightly differing alignments.

As interesting specimens for material scientists, strained or stressed polymer samples were inspected. In Figure 10, a polymer sheet exhibiting known external or internal defects is shown, examined by PS-OCT during a stretching process. In the intensity-based OCT image, defects are slightly recognizable, but the fringe pattern in the retardation image point to defects through the deviations from the regular pattern. By applying increasing stress, the evolution of the fringes can be observed over time. The progression of fringe frequency over imaging depth or time correlates with the formation of internal stress and strain fields.

Through subsequent image processing and under consideration of optical material constants, a quantitative analysis of strain based on the retardation fringe pattern can be performed [50].

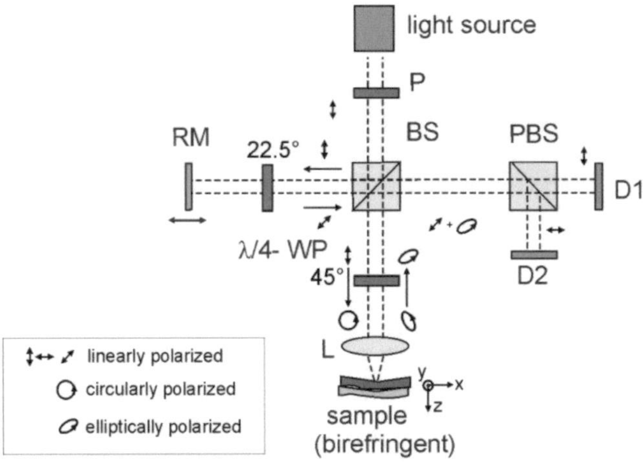

Figure 9. The optical (time domain) PS-OCT setup (Michelson configuration) containing additionally polarizing optical elements (WP: wave plate, P: polarizer, PBS: polarizing beam splitter) for a dual channel detection (D1, D2).

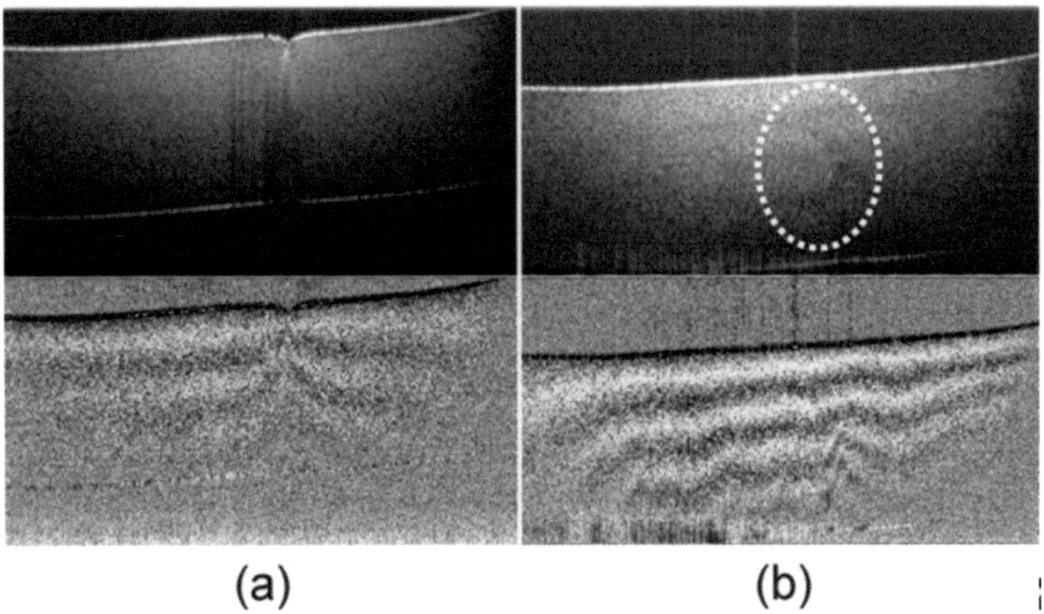

Figure 10. Strained polymer sample (thickness 1mm) under increasing tensile load under PS-OCT imaging shown as intensity cross-sections (upper images) and corresponding gray-scale encoded retardation images (bottom images): (a) sample exhibiting a surface defect, (b) sample with internal defect (visible as slightly darker, bow-shaped feature within marked region). Reprinted from [46], with permission from OSA, © 2010.

Another interesting example of PS imaging concerns the investigation of micro-structured polymer materials [51], represented here by a semi-transparent polymer mould for micromechanical wheels, to gain insight into hidden stress states resulting from the manufacturing and from the subsequent curing processes. In Figure 11, the en-face reflectivity and retardation image of the micro-component is shown, which was probed under a transversal scanning scheme by means of PS-OCT imaging.

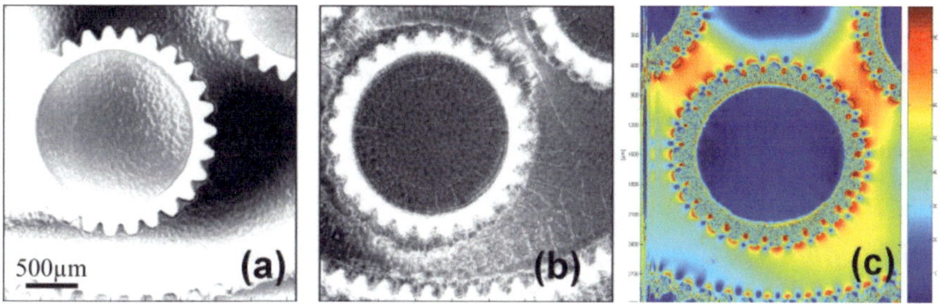

Figure 11. Micro-structured polymer part (photoresist mould for a micromechanical wheel, thickness 1.5 mm) imaged by PS-OCT [51]. The intensity-based reflectivity images are shown at surface (a) and backside (b), and the corresponding retardation image (c). Larger areas of regions with induced strain fields are visible between the wheels; smaller stressed regions appear between the teeth.

A similar region imaged by PS-FF-OCM is depicted in Figure 12. For the FF-OCM, an increased scattering in the polymer part is remarkable compared to OCT, (illumination: SLD).

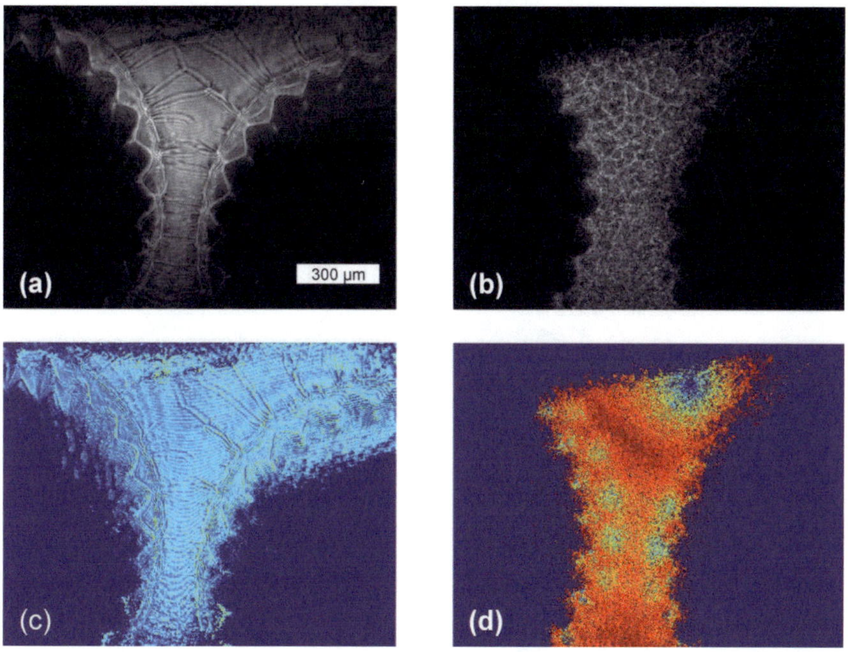

Figure 12. Micro-structured polymer part (section of photoresist mould) imaged by PS-FF-OCM. The intensity-based reflectivity images at surface (a) and backside (b), and the corresponding retardation images (c) and (d). Note smaller regions with local stress-strain fields between the teeth (d).

As a further application for PS-OCT, we briefly mention the in-situ monitoring of crystallization processes during the extrusion, shearing, and solidification of the polymer material [52]. The growing of polymer micro-crystallites and the evolution of different planar polymer structures during the processes can be visualized by PS-OCT and be analyzed with respect to the process parameters (temperature, pressure, speed). The resulting micro-crystalline structures within the polymer matrix are monitored by (PS)-FF-OCM imaging with a higher lateral resolution (compared to PS-OCT) as depicted in Figure 13. The different edges of the crystallite are clearly visible in the intensity-based full-field images. Furthermore, an optical anisotropy of the crystallites can be observed in the retardation images of the polarization sensitive full-field version.

Other PS-OCT or PS-FF-OCM imaging applications in a technical context concern ceramics [53], fiber-reinforced polymer compounds [54], or organic coatings [55]. However, without doubt the main application field for PS-OCT and PS-FF-OCM is still that of numerous medical applications. [56, 57].

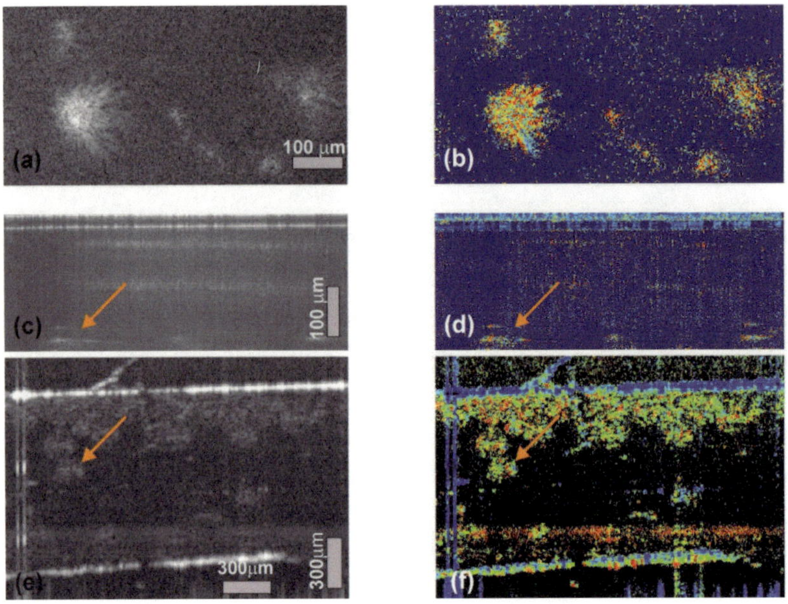

Figure 13. Visualization of micro-crystalline structures in isotactic polypropylene grown during the extrusion and crystallization process. (a) and (c) reflectivity images, (b) and (d) retardation images obtained by PS-FF-OCM. The images are depicted as en-face image (upper row) and as cross-section (middle row). For comparison: reflectivity (e) and retardation cross-sectional scans (f) of the entire polymer sample, examined by PS-OCT imaging. The arrows indicate micro-crystallites in both cross-sectional images (PS-FF-OCM and PS-OCT). Note the different fields of view in OCT and FF-OCM imaging.

http://dx.doi.org/10.5772/53509

4.4. Contrast modification in FF-OCM imaging

Additional to the issues of obtaining suitable resolution and focus depth in microscopy imaging, an appropriate contrast enhancement or modification is essential to emphasis special features of the specimen. Similar to configurations in microscopy, in FF-OCM different contrast modifications can be realized. Based on the traditional principle of Fourier plane filtering, a Fourier filter unit is incorporated into the FF-OCM setup, preferably as a Mach-Zehnder configuration. The Fourier filter unit comprehends a 4f configuration, depicted schematically in Figure 14. The key element is the optical Fourier filter in the back-focal plane of the entrance lens. Whereas in the past, the optical filter was often manufactured as a silica or glass component, the filter can nowadays be realized by a spatial light modulator (SLM) [58].

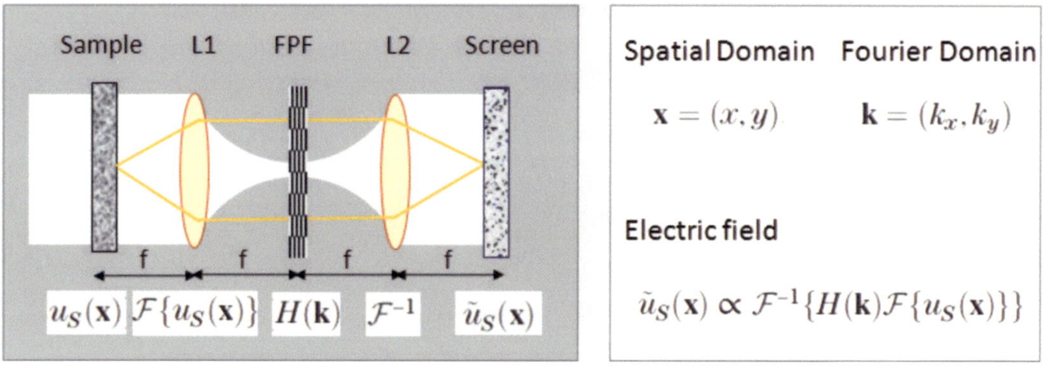

Figure 14. Illustration scheme of the optical Fourier filtering principle. The 4f-configuration is depicted in the left panel. It consists of the sample, entrance lens (L1), Fourier filter (FPF), exit lens (L2), and reconstructed object recorded at the screen. Each component is positioned at a distance to the focal length f from one another. The mathematical terms are given in the right panel: forward and inverse Fourier transform (F and F^{-1}) and filter function *H*(k) applied to sample wave function u_s(x) results in a modified wave field $\tilde{u}_s$(x).

The SLM, as a pixelated liquid crystal array, is addressable with different amplitude or phase filter functions. The contrast can now be changed flexibly and be adapted to the sample [59]. Similar to microscopy, phase contrast, Schlieren contrast, or spiral phase contrast are emulated to enhance partial sites of the imaged structure (Figure 15). But in contrast to microscopy imaging, the contrast modification in FF-OCM can now be performed in a depth-resolved way (Figure 16).

Fourier plane filters In FF-OCM are most useful for imaging stratified or layered, almost transparent samples like varnish coatings or droplets. It should be mentioned that for highly scattering materials, phase-based Fourier filtering may fail because no fixed phase relation can be build up between the random scatters. Here, a novel method for focusing light through scattering materials seems a promising approach [60, 61].

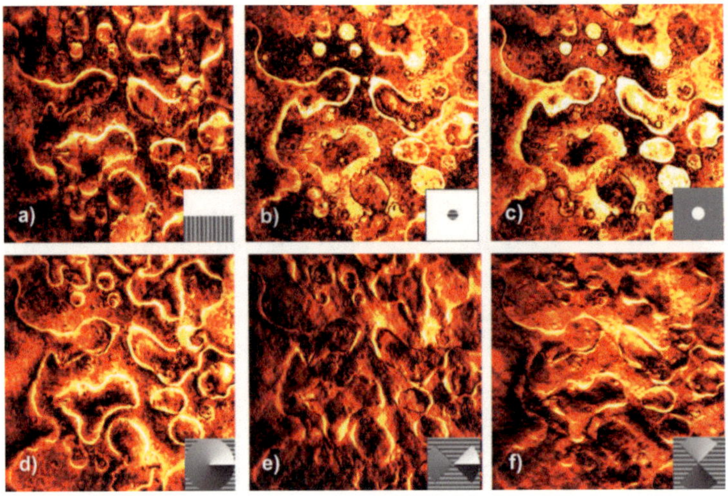

Figure 15. Illustration of flexible contrast in FF-OCM imaging on a test sample (organic varnish droplets applied to both the front and back surface of a glass slide, mimicking a multilayered technical structure). The emulated contrast comprehends (a) dark field contrast, (b) Schlieren contrast, (c) phase contrast, (d) isotropic spiral-phase contrast, and (e), (f) anisotropic contrast with cone-like spiral phase filters. A pseudo-colour representation is chosen. The applied FPFs are indicated schematically in the insets. Reprinted from [59], with permission from GIT Verlag.

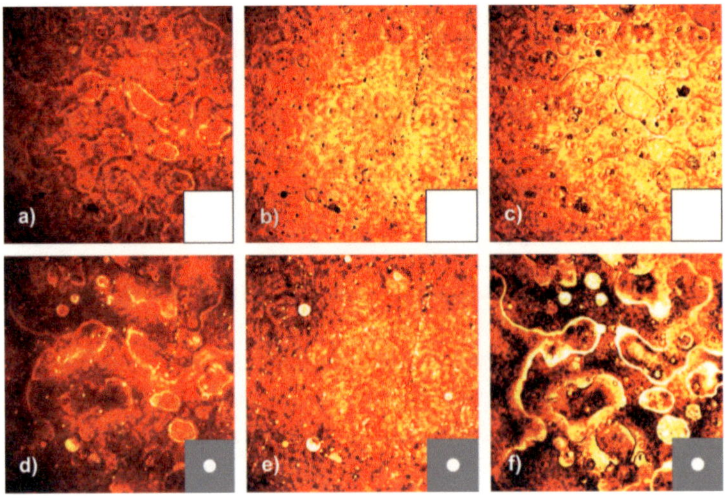

Figure 16. Comparison of depth-selective contrast modification in microscopic and FF-OCM imaging, exemplified for a varnish droplet test sample. The features are visualized in (a) and (d) by conventional microscopy, in (b), (c), (e), and (f) by OCM imaging; the scans are taken at the upper ((b) and (e)), and lower interface ((c) and (f)) of the test sample. First row: bright field mode; second row: phase contrast mode. Reprinted from [59], with permission from GIT Verlag.

5. Conclusions and outlook

We have demonstrated different applications of FF-OCM in the field of material sciences, with a particular focus on examples from polymer sciences. FF-OCM is a promising non-destructive technique for the investigation of novel polymer materials, in particular if local distribution of fibers and filler particles should be monitored or combined with polarization-sensitive versions if local stress states are of interest. Furthermore, we have illustrated how adapted image processing can further contribute to a better extraction of the information contained in OCT and OCM images. It should be mentioned that in diverse applications, OCT and FF-OCM measurements may supplement each other by providing partly complementary information due to their different resolution and penetration abilities.

Although literature about OCT and FF-OCM applications in material research is in the minority compared to applications in the medical field, we hope that newly established dialogue between these two research areas and the increase of interest on the side of material scientists to take up novel techniques may continue into future.

Acknowledgements

The financial support by the Federal Ministry of Economy, Family and Youth, the National Foundation for Research, Technology and Development is gratefully acknowledged. For the micro-CT measurements on SGF-PP samples, we thank Dietmar Salaberger and Bernhard Plank at the Applied University of Upper Austria, Wels. Furthermore, we are grateful to Prof. Heide at the TU Bergakademie Freiberg for providing the mineral specimens, Peter Hierzenberger and Roman Rittberger at Polymer Sciences Department, JKU Linz for preparing the different polymer materials. We acknowledge Prof. Ritsch-Marte and team at the Medical University Innsbruck for continuous support in SLM techniques. Jean-Luc Bouchot at JKU Linz and Sören Häuser at the University Kaiserslautern are given thanks for their contributions in image processing.

Author details

Bettina Heise[1,2*], Stefan Schausberger[1] and David Stifter[1]

*Address all correspondence to: Bettina.Heise@jku.at

1 Christian Doppler Laboratory for Microscopic and Spectroscopic Material Characterization, Johannes Kepler University, Linz, Austria

2 FLLL, Johannes Kepler University, Linz, Austria

References

[1] Harrer B, Kastner J. X-ray microtomography: Characterization of structures and defect analysis, In: Fabrication and Characterization in the Micro-Nano Range, A. Lasagni, F. Lasagni (Publ.), Vol 10, Springer Verlag, Heidelberg, 2011. p119-149. doi 10.1007/978-3-642-17782-8.

[2] Huang D, Swanson EA, Lin CP, Schuman JS, Stinson WG, Chang W, Hee MR, Flotte T, Gregory K, Puliafito CA, Fujimo JG. Optical Coherence Tomography, Science 1991; 254 (5035), 1178–1181.

[3] Fercher AF, Sander B, Jorgensen TM, Andersen PE. Optical Coherence Tomography. Encyclopedia of Analytic Chemistry 2009.

[4] Li N, Zhang S, Hou J, Jang IK, Yu B. Assessment of Pulmonary Artery Morphology by Optical Coherence Tomography. Heart Lung Circ. 2012; in press, online August 2012.

[5] Payton S. Kidney cancer: First in vivo study shows optical imaging can distinguish renal cancer from normal tissue. Nat. Rev. Urol. 2012; 9(6), 294.

[6] Shlivko IL, Petrova GA, Zorkina MV, Tchekalkina OE, Firsova MS, Ellinsky DO, Agrba PD, Kamensky VA, Donchenko EV. Complex assessment of age-specific morphofunctional features of skin of different anatomic localizations. Skin Research and Technology, in press, online June 2012.

[7] Park HC, Song C, Kang M, Jeong Y, Jeong KH. Forward imaging OCT endoscopic catheter based on MEMS lens scanning, Opt. Lett. 2012; 37(13), 2673-2675

[8] Davidson M, Kaufmann K, Mazor I, Cohen F. An application of interference microscopy to integrated circuit inspection and metrology. SPIE 1987; Proc. 775, 233-241.

[9] Liang H, Lawman S. High precision dynamic multi-interface profilometry with optical coherence tomography. Appl. Optics 2011; 50(32), 6039-6048.

[10] Yang ML, Winkler AM, Klein J, Wall A, Barton JK. Using Optical Coherence Tomography to Characterize the Crack Morphology of Ceramic Glaze and Jade. In: Selected Topics in Optical Coherence Tomography. Intech, online: doi: 10.5772/31213.

[11] Prykäri T, Czajkowski J, Alarousu E, Myllylä R. Optical coherence tomography as an accurate inspection and quality evaluation technique in paper industry. Opt. Rev. 2010; 17(3), 218-222.

[12] Webster PJL, Yu JXZ, Leung BYC, Anderson MD, Yang VXD, Fraser JM. In situ 24 kHz coherent imaging of morphology change in laser percussion drilling. Opt. Lett. 2010; 35(5), 646-648.

[13] Stifter D. Beyond biomedicine: a review of alternative applications and developments for optical coherence tomography. Appl. Phys. 2007; 88, 337-479.

[14] Xi C, Marks DL, Parikh DS, Raskin L, Boppart SA. Structural and functional imaging of 3D microfluidic mixers using optical coherence tomography. PNAS 2004; 101(20), 7516-7521.

[15] Stifter D, Burgholzer P, Höglinger O, Götzinger E, Hitzenberger CK. Polarisation-sensitive optical coherence tomography for material characterisation and strain-field mapping. Appl. Phys. A 2003; 76(6), 947-951.

[16] Wieser W, Biedermann BR, Klein T, Eigenwillig CM, Huber R. Multi-Mega-hertz OCT: High quality 3D imaging at 20 million A-scans and 4.5 GVoxels per second. Opt.Express 2010; 18(14), 14685-14704.

[17] Sun J, Xie H. MEMS-Based Endoscopic Optical Coherence Tomography. Inter. J. Optics 2011; ID 825629, online: doi:10.1155/2011/825629.

[18] Ju MJ, Lee SJ, Kim Y, Shin SG, Kim HY, Lim Y, Yasuno Y, Lee BH. Multimodal analysis of pearls and pearl treatments by using optical coherence tomography and fluorescence spectroscopy. Opt. Express 2011; 19(7), 6420-6432.

[19] Skala MC, Fontanella A, Hendargo H, Dewhirst MW, Izatt, JA, Combined Hyperspectral and Spectral Domain Optical Coherence Tomography Microscope for Non-invasive Hemodynamic Imaging. Opt. Lett. 2009; 34(3), 289-291.

[20] Liu G, Chen Z. Fiber-based combined optical coherence and multiphoton endomicroscopy. J Biomed Opt. 2011, 16(3), 036010-1-4.

[21] Graf BW. Multimodal in vivo skin imaging with integrated optical coherence and multiphoton microscopy. IEEE J. Selected Topics in Quantum Electronics 2012; 18(4), 1280-1286.

[22] Dubois A, Vabre L, Boccara AC, Beaurepaire E. High-Resolution Full-Field Optical Coherence Tomography with a Linnik Microscope. Appl. Opt. 2002; 41(4), 805-812.

[23] Fang L, Li S, Nie Q, Izatt JA, Toth CA, Farsiu S. Sparsity Based Denoising of Spectral Domain Optical Coherence Tomography Images. Biomed. Opt. Express, 3(5), 927-942.

[24] Huang Y, Liu X, Kang JU. Real-time 3D and 4D Fourier domain Doppler optical coherence tomography based on dual graphics processing units. Biomed. Opt. Express 2012; 13(9), 2162-2174.

[25] Dubois A, Boccara AC. Full-Field Optical Coherence Tomography. In: Drexler W, Fujimoto JF (eds.) Optical Coherence Tomography. Springer; 2008. p565-591.

[26] Bayleyegn MD, Makhlouf H, Crotti C, Plamann K, Dubois A, Ultrahigh resolution spectral-domain optical coherence tomography at 1.3 μm using a broadband super-luminescent diode light source. Opt. Commun. 2012, in press, online August 2012, dx.doi.org/10.1016/j.optcom.2012.07.066.

[27] Wiesauer K. Pircher M, Götzinger E, Bauer S, Engelke R, Ahrens G, Grützner G, Hitzenberger CK, Stifter D. En-face scanning optical coherence tomography with ultra-high resolution for material investigation. Opt. Express 2005; 13 (3), 1015-1024.

[28] Hartl I, Li XD, Chudoba C, Ghanta RK, Ko TH, Fujimoto JG, Ranka JK, Windeler RS. Ultrahigh-resolution optical coherence tomography using continuum generation in an air–silica microstructure optical fiber. Opt. Lett. 2001; 26, 608-610.

[29] Humbert G, Wadsworth WJ, Leon-Saval SG, Knight JC, Birks TA, Russell PSJ, Lederer MJ, Kopf D, Wiesauer K, Breuer EI, Stifter D. Supercontinuum generation system for optical coherence tomography based on tapered photonic crystal fibre. Opt. Express 2006; 14 (4), 1596-1603.

[30] Dubois A, Grieve K, Moneron G, Lecaque R, Vabre L, Boccara C. Ultrahigh- resolution full-field optical coherence tomography. Appl. Opt. 2004; 43, 2874–2883.

[31] Heise B, Schausberger SE, Häuser S, Plank B, Salaberger D, Leiss-Holzinger E, Stifter D. Full-Field Optical Coherence Microscopy with a Sub-nanosecond Supercontinuum Light Source for Material Research. Opt. Fiber Technol. 2012, in press, dx.doi.org/10.1016/j.yofte.2012.07.011.

[32] Adachi M. Phase-shift algorithm for white-light interferometry insensitive to a linear error in phase shift increment. 2005; Proc. SPIE 6048, 604806-1-9.

[33] Malacara D, Servin M, Malacara Z. Inteferogram Analysis for Optical Testing. CRC Press, Taylor& Francis Group (2005). p475-491.

[34] Hrebesh MS. Full-Field & Single-Shot Full-Field Optical Coherence Tomography: A novel technique for biomedical imaging applications. Advances in Optical Technologies 2012 (2012); ID 435408, online: doi:10.1155/2012/435408.

[35] Bernstein S, Bouchot, JL Reinhardt M, Heise B. Generalized Analytic Signals in Image Processing: Comparison, Theory and Applications. TIM Birkhäuser, accepted 2012.

[36] Hahn SL. Multi-dimensional complex signals with single-orthant spectra. Proc. IEEE 1992; 80, 1287-1300.

[37] Felsberg M, Sommer G. The monogenic signal. IEEE Trans. Sign. Proc. 2001; 49(12), 3136-3144.

[38] Larkin KG, Bone DJ, Oldfield MA. Natural demodulation of two-dimensional fringe patterns. I. General background of the spiral phase quadrature transform. J. Opt. Soc. Am. A 2001; 18(8), 1862-1870.

[39] Nugroho W, Hrebesh MS, Sato M. Simulation of basic characteristics of single-shot full-field optical coherence tomography using spatially phase-modulated reference light. Opt. Rev. 2011; 18(4), 343-350.

[40] Hrebesh MS, Dabu R, Sato M. In vivo imaging of dynamic biological specimen by real-time single-shot full-field optical coherence tomography. Opt. Commun. 2009; 282, 674-683.

[41] Razani M, Mariampillai A, Sun C, Luk TW, Yang VX, Kolios MC. Feasibility of optical coherence elastography measurements of shear wave propagation in homogeneous tissue equivalent phantoms. Biomed. Opt. Express 2012; 3(5), 972-980.

[42] Adie SG, Liang X, Kennedy BF, John R, Sampson DD, Boppart SA. Spectroscopic optical coherence elastography. Opt. Express 2010; 18(25), 25519-25534.

[43] Schlager V, Schausberger SE, Stifter D, Heise B. Coherence probe microscopy imaging and analysis for fiber-reinforced polymers. Springer LNCS 2011; 6688, 424-434.

[44] Häuser S. Fast Finite Shearlet Transform: a tutorial. Preprint University of Kaiserslautern, 2011, arXiv:1202.1773v1.

[45] Unser M, Sage D, Van De Ville D. Multiresolution monogenic signal analysis using the Riesz-Laplace wavelet transform, IEEE Trans. Image Proc. 2009; 18(11), 2402-2418.

[46] Stifter D, Leiss-Holzinger E, Major Z, Baumann B, Pircher M, Götzinger E, Hitzenberger CK, Heise B. Dynamic optical studies in materials testing with spectral-domain polarization-sensitive optical coherence tomography. Opt. Express 2010; 18(25), 25712-25725.

[47] Schausberger SE, Heise B, Bernstein S, Stifter D. Full-field optical coherence microscopy with a sCMOS detector for dynamic imaging, Opt. Lett., submitted.

[48] Baumann B, Baumann SO, Konegger T, Pircher M, Götzinger E, Schlanitz F. et al. Polarization sensitive optical coherence tomography of melanin provides intrinsic contrast based on depolarization. Biomed. Opt. Express 2012; 3(7), 1670-1683.

[49] Moneron G, Boccara AC, Dubois A. Polarization-sensitive full-field optical coherence tomography. Opt. Lett. 2007; 32(14), 2058-2060.

[50] Heise B, Wiesauer K, Götzinger E, Pircher M, Hitzenberger CK, Engelke R, Ahrens G, Grützner G, Stifter D. Spatially Resolved Stress Measurements in Materials with Polarisation-Sensitive Optical Coherence Tomography: Image Acquisition and Processing Aspects. J. Strain 2010; 46, 61-68.

[51] Wiesauer K, Pircher M, Götzinger E, Hitzenberger CK, Engelke R, Ahrens G, Grützner G, Stifter D. Transversal ultrahigh-resolution polarization-sensitive optical coherence tomography for strain mapping in materials. Opt. Express 2006; 14, 5945-5953.

[52] Hierzenberger P, Eder G, Heise B, Leiss-Holzinger E, Stifter D. In-situ monitoring of polymer crystallization by Optical Coherence Tomography (OCT). Proc. Advances in Polymer Science and Technology 2, Trauner Verlag, Linz 2011.

[53] Strakowski M, Pluciński J, Łoziński A, Kosmowski BB. Determination of local polarization properties of PLZT ceramics by PS-OCT. The European Physical Journal - Special Topics 2008; 154(1), 207-210.

[54] Wiesauer K, Pircher M, Götzinger E, Hitzenberger CK, Oster R, Stifter D. Investigation of glass–fibre reinforced polymers by polarisation-sensitive, ultra-high resolution optical coherence tomography: Internal structures, defects and stress. Composites Science and Technology 2007; 67(15-16), 3051–3058.

[55] Dubois A. Spectroscopic polarization-sensitive full-field optical coherence tomography. Opt. Express 2012; 20(9), 9962-9977.

[56] Kang H, Darling CL, Fried D. Nondestructive monitoring of the repair of enamel artificial lesions by an acidic remineralization model using polarization-sensitive optical coherence tomography. Dental Materials 2012; 28(5), 488-494.

[57] Baumann B, Pircher M, Götzinger E, Sattmann H, Wurm M, Stifter D, Schütze C, Ahlers C, Geitzenauer W, Schmidt-Erfurth U, Hitzenberger CK. Imaging the human retina in vivo with combined spectral-domain polarization-sensitive optical coherence tomography and scanning laser ophtalmoscopy. SPIE 2009; Proc. 7163; 71630N-1-6.

[58] Maurer C, Jesacher A, Bernet S, Ritsch-Marte M. What spatial light modulators can do for optical microscopy. Laser & Photonics Reviews 2011; 5(1), 81-101.

[59] Heise B, Schausberger SE, Stifter D. Coherence Probe Microscopy Contrast Modification and Image Enhancement. Imaging & Microscopy 2012; 2, 29-32.

[60] Vellekoop IM, Mosk AP. Focusing coherent light through opaque strongly scattering media.Opt. Lett. 2007; 32(16), 2309-2311.

[61] Stockbridge C, Lu Y, Moore J, Hoffman S, Paxman R, Toussaint K, Bifano T. Focusing through dynamic scattering media. Opt. Express 2012; 20(14), 15086-15092.

Chapter 9

Optical Coherence Tomography – Applications in Non-Destructive Testing and Evaluation

Alexandra Nemeth, Günther Hannesschläger, Elisabeth Leiss-Holzinger, Karin Wiesauer and Michael Leitner

Additional information is available at the end of the chapter

http://dx.doi.org/10.5772/53960

1. Introduction

The field of non-destructive testing and evaluation (NDTE) comprises many different techniques and approaches. Over the past few decades there have been tremendous advances in NDTE technology, allowing researchers and engineers to tackle problems in many scientific and industrial fields. However, techniques enabling a fast, contactless, non-invasive, and high-resolution imaging of subsurface features at a level of only a few microns are still scarce.

One technology fulfilling all of these requirements is optical coherence tomography (OCT) [1]. OCT is a purely optical, non-destructive, non-invasive, and contactless high resolution imaging method, which allows the acquisition of one-, two- or three-dimensional depth resolved image data of sub-surface regions in situ and in real time. The outstanding depth resolution of OCT can be as good as or even better than one micrometer [2]. OCT is an already well-established diagnostics technique for biomedicine and advanced life science applications. Emerging originally from the field of ophthalmology, OCT has also received a lot of interest in other biomedical areas like e.g. dentistry [3], dermatology [4], cardiology [5], and developmental biology [6].

The potential of OCT to become an outstanding imaging technique also outside the area of biomedicine has been recognized already within the first years after its invention [7,8]. However, only a few groups applied the technology to material related problems, and therefore the interest for this field of research has increased slowly [9–12]. A comprehensive review on OCT applications outside biomedicine was published by Stifter in 2007 [13].

Since then OCT has received increasing attention as a novel tool for NDTE, with more and more research groups being engaged in further exploring possible applications of OCT. Recent examples include, among many others, the measurement of layer thickness in multi-layered foils [14] or pharmaceutical tablets [15], the characterization of laser-drilled holes and micro-machined devices [16], organic solar cells [17], paper [18], or printed electronics products [19], applications in food [20] and polymer sciences [21], and the conservation of artwork [22].

This chapter will give a short overview on the technique of OCT, provide a brief overview on the historical development of OCT for non-destructive testing, and describe some of the most recent applications in this field.

2. Optical coherence tomography

OCT is based on the physical phenomenon of white light interferometry (WLI) and employs special light sources with high spatial but low temporal coherence (i.e., a large bandwidth spectrum), like e.g. superluminescent diodes, or femtosecond or supercontinuum lasers. Such sources have coherence lengths in the range of only several microns. In an interferometric detection system such a short coherence length acts like a temporal filter regarding the arrival times of the back-scattered photons. For currently used low coherence light sources the coherence length generally lies in the region of 1-15 μm, enabling an excellent axial (depth) resolution with OCT [2]. Due to the interferometric detection scheme OCT is well suited to image layered and micro-structured samples. The image contrast is due to inhomogeneities in the refractive index of the sample material, and thus, OCT provides complementary information to other high resolution imaging techniques like ultrasound, X-ray computed tomography (CT), and magnetic resonance imaging (MRI).

The nomenclature in OCT is analogous to the one used in ultrasound tomography. Single depth scans and cross-sections are classified as A- and B-scans, respectively. When imaging at a constant depth, it is possible to acquire the so-called en-face images or C-scans. The image plane of C-scans is perpendicular to the one of B-scans and has the familiar orientation of conventional microscopy images. An M-scan describes the acquisition of consecutive A-scans at one constant lateral position. In this case one dimension in the 2D image represents the progress in time.

2.1. Resolution

In comparison to other high resolution microscopic techniques, like e.g. confocal microscopy, OCT has the advantage that axial and lateral resolutions are decoupled. Therefore the imaging optics can be located away from the sample without penalizing the axial resolution. The axial resolution is limited by the center wavelength and the bandwidth of the optical light source, and is generally defined as one half of the coherence length l_c:

http://dx.doi.org/10.5772/53960

$$\Delta z = \frac{l_c}{2} = K\frac{\lambda_c^2}{\Delta\lambda}. \tag{1}$$

Here K denotes a constant factor (0.44 for an optical source with Gaussian spectral distribution), and λ_c and $\Delta\lambda$ describe the center wavelength and full width at half maximum (FWHM) bandwidth of the source, respectively.

The lateral resolution is solely determined by the probe optics and can be calculated over

$$\Delta x = 0.61\frac{\lambda}{NA} \tag{2}$$

where NA is the numerical aperture of the imaging optics.

2.2. Spectral range and light sources

In OCT the sample is commonly illuminated with light in the near infrared (NIR). The choice of the right light source is crucial since it determines on the one hand the axial resolution and on the other hand the penetration depth. Light sources used in OCT should have very high spatial but very low temporal coherence (i.e. a large spectral bandwidth) and provide a smooth Gaussian shaped spectrum. In this way axial resolutions in the range of one micrometer can be achieved.

The penetration depth is determined by the attenuation characteristics of the sample, which can be described by the Beer-Lambert law

$$I_D(\lambda, z) = I_0 R_z \exp\left\{-2\int_0^z \mu_{att}(\lambda, z')dz'\right\} \tag{3}$$

where I_D describes the intensity measured at the detector, I_0 the initial intensity, R_z the reflection coefficient at depth z, and μ_{att} the attenuation coefficient. The attenuation coefficient μ_{att} is the sum of the scattering and the absorption coefficients, μ_{sca} and μ_{abs}, respectively, which are both functions of the wavelength λ. Consequently, the penetration depth is strongly dependent on the wavelength range used for the imaging process, since this determines the absorption and scattering of the light. With the right choice of the light source penetration depths of several millimeters can be achieved.

Historically the most important application for OCT is ophthalmology. Therefore a great part of the commercially available OCT systems are designed towards this specific application and comprise light sources centered around 800 nm, where absorption due to water is low. For many non-ophthalmic applications, however, it has been shown that imaging at different center wavelengths might be advantageous [13]. Promising spectral regions are located around 1300 nm and 1550 nm. Here scattering is reduced for many samples and the penetration depth is drastically increased. Anyway, the technique of OCT is applicable on a vast variety of materials, and basically for every application the most suitable spectral range has to be determined.

The three types of light sources mostly used in OCT are superluminescence diodes, femtosecond lasers, and supercontinuum laser sources. Since superluminescence diodes are rather cheap, provide nicely shaped Gaussian spectra, and are available at many different center wavelengths, they are the most popular kind of light source for OCT. However, the FWHM bandwidth of superluminescence diodes is limited to ≈ 100 nm, which constrains the axial resolution to several micrometers. Femtosecond laser sources offer higher bandwidths (typically up to ≈ 200 nm) and increased optical power, but are relatively expensive. Supercontinuum laser sources can cover a spectrum ranging from around 400 nm to 2400 nm, allowing for the acquisition of ultra-high resolution images.

2.3. Image acquisition and detection schemes

OCT is an interferometric approach, in which the depth-resolved information can be assessed by different means. In all approaches the probing beam is focused into the object and photons are back-scattered from different sample structures like interfaces, impurities, pores or cells. Only single scattered photons contribute to the useful signal, and by comparing their arrival times with a reference light beam a depth scan is obtained. Reconstruction of depth resolved cross sections (2D images) or volumes (3D images) is performed by scanning the probing beam laterally across the sample with the aid of galvanometer mirrors and subsequent acquisition of depth scans at adjacent lateral positions.

The depth resolved OCT signal can be acquired either in the time-domain or the spectral-domain, with the latter approach offering advantages in terms of imaging speed and sensitivity, enabling video rate imaging [23] and in-line applications [14]. On the other hand, the time-domain approach permits dynamic focusing and shows a constant sensitivity over the whole depth range.

In time-domain OCT the length of the reference arm in the interferometer is scanned over several millimeters while the sample is kept static. Due to the interferometric detection scheme and the short coherence length of the used light sources, a signal is detected only if the photons reflected from both interferometer arms have travelled the same optical distance to the photodetector. Otherwise only noise is detected. Obviously, the mechanical movement of the reference mirror is rather time consuming and may lead to mechanical instabilities and noise.

One way to speed up the image acquisition process is to use the so-called Fourier-domain OCT approach. Here the reference mirror is fixed and the light coming from both reference and object is detected in a spectrally resolved way. This can either be done in parallel (spectral-domain) by using a dispersing element and a CCD or CMOS camera, or sequentially by scanning a narrow laser line over a broad spectral region (swept-source OCT). Whatever the approach, in Fourier-domain OCT the depth information is encoded in a cosinusoidal modulation of the acquired spectrum and can be accessed by applying an inverse Fourier transform. With state-of-the-art cameras or swept laser sources A-scan rates of several hundred kHz can be achieved.

A schematic of a spectral-domain OCT system (left), and a photograph of an industrial OCT system, as developed in the labs at RECENDT (right), are depicted in Figure 1.

http://dx.doi.org/10.5772/53960

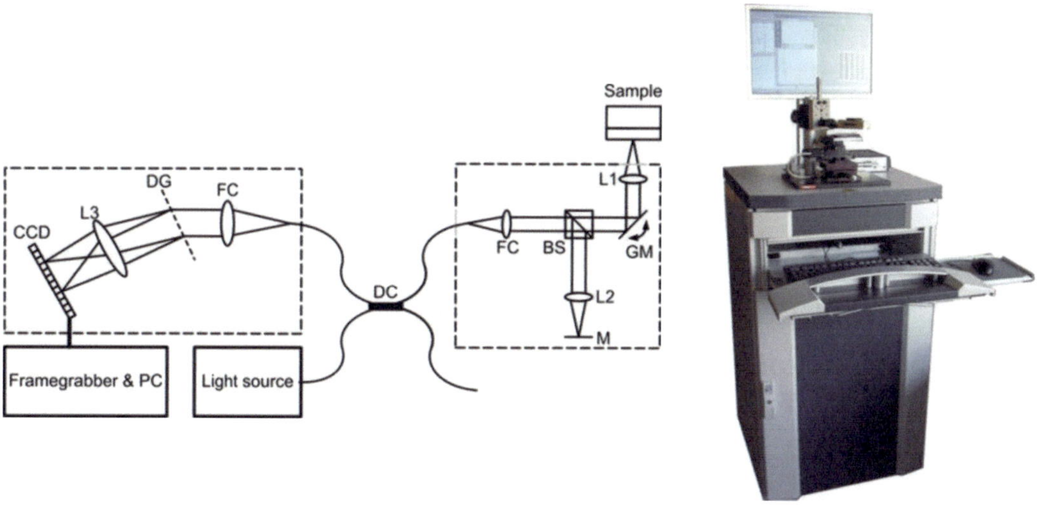

Figure 1. Left: Schematic of a spectral-domain OCT system. The dashed boxes represent portable and independent modules. DC – directional coupler; FC – fibre coupler; BS – beamsplitter; (G)M – (galvanometer) mirror; LX – lens; DG – diffraction grating. Right: Photograph of a spectral-domain OCT system developed at RECENDT.

3. Applications of OCT in non-destructive testing

OCT can provide both quantitative and qualitative information. The former includes e.g. the thickness of layers, or the size and distribution of pores, fibers or cells. With the aid of state-of-the-art image processing tools it is possible to automatically analyze sample features. Qualitative information is obtained through the visual inspection of the acquired images. Features like surfaces, impurities or cells can easily be detected and give rapid indications on the condition of the sample, providing important information to scientists or technicians.

Besides sample information based on pure reflectivity, it is also possible to take advantage of other types of contrast like birefringence for the detection of stress and strain (polarization-sensitive OCT) [12], the direction and velocity of fluids (Doppler OCT) [24], and spectral characteristics (spectroscopic or differential absorption OCT) [25].

Generally, information on the sample under investigation by means of OCT can be acquired under three different conditions: (i) with a lab based system assembled on an optical bench, (ii) with a desktop system (e.g. a commercially available device or a prototype system like in Figure 1), or (iii) directly at a production site in an industrial environment. Therefore, for each application the right system has to be chosen.

Lab-based systems have the most degrees of freedom, since different components like appropriate light sources, scanners, and detection devices can easily be connected in order to enable a rapid investigation of the sample. The drawback of such systems is that they are confined to the optical bench where all devices are assembled.

Nowadays there already exist several companies and research centers offering commercially available OCT systems or prototypes, respectively, which aim at applications outside the medical sector and the common optics laboratory. Generally, in such OCT devices all the necessary components, mostly except the computer, are embedded in one single casing. Such systems are ideal for test measurements and to analyze many kinds of samples. However, desktop systems offer little degrees of freedom, albeit several suppliers offer the possibility to built custom-inspired systems.

In some cases there is the need to tailor OCT systems towards one particular application. In biomedical imaging (e.g. ophthalmology, dermatology) this is already common practice. In the field of NDTE, however, there is still a quest for the "killer application", which would trigger the development of commercially available OCT systems tailored towards the investigation of one particular kind of sample. Therefore, so far most of the OCT systems used for the characterization of processes or specimens at industrial sites are specially designed prototypes, which hence are also still quite expensive. Recently one promising application coming up was the in-line-characterization of multi-layered foils directly at the production site [14].

The remainder of this chapter is now dedicated to the discussion of some recent applications of OCT in the field of non-destructive testing.

3.1. Characterization of multi-layered foils

Multi-layered plastic foils are commonly employed in the packaging industry to preserve the content from environmental influences. In food packaging, for example, different layers fulfill different purposes, such as protecting the interior from oxygen or providing good vapor permeability from the inside out. The production process of multi-layered foils at blown film extrusion lines typically comprises only one step. Especially in the case of barrier layers it is very important to guarantee the right layer thickness. The material used for such barrier layers is expensive, and therefore any material used in excess turns the production less cost-effective. On the other hand, if the layer is too thin the specifications might not be met, turning the foil useless. In order to ensure already during the production process that the final product matches the specifications, an in-line quality control is required. The parameters that need to be monitored in-line include the thickness and homogeneity of the individual layers and possible inclusions of air or impurities. A method to perform this task has to be non-destructive, fast, and must provide the ability to reveal the internal structure of (semi-)transparent media.

Typically the overall foil thickness is measured in-line by radiographic means. This approach, however, uses hazardous radiation and does not enable the determination of the thickness of the individual layers. This parameter is usually controlled over the weight of the foil material before entering the blown film extrusion line. So far, a reliable control of the final product, however, is only performed off-line. To this end samples pieces are cut out of the multi-layered foils and are analyzed by destructive means, like e.g. microtome microscopy. This approach is time consuming and the results are only available several hours after the production of the foil. Therefore, during this time period the quality of the foil is unknown and it is well possible that the whole intermediate production has to be classified as waste.

The non-destructive and contactless nature of OCT turns this technique an ideal tool for the analysis and quality control of multi-layered foils and other coated structures, as they are often used in the packaging industry. Films with a thickness of only a few microns can easily be resolved with common OCT systems, therefore enabling the analysis of film thickness homogeneity and the detection of impurities [11]. With knowledge on the refractive index of the single layers in the multi-layered foils, even an exact measure of the sample thickness can be provided. With fast OCT systems it is possible to monitor the thickness of the individual layers in moving foils or even in-line [14].

To test the feasibility of OCT to image multi-layered foils moving at different speeds some first off-line tests were performed at the facilities of RECENDT. The experiments were conducted with a portable high speed and high resolution spectral-domain OCT system, similar to the one presented in Figure 1. To meet the requirements of the experiment, the system was equipped with a specially designed single point probing head. A detailed description of the system can be found in [14]. Generally, OCT cross section images are obtained by scanning the probing beam across the sample. In this special application, however, the sample already moves at high speeds in the lateral direction, enabling therefore the acquisition of depth scans at different lateral positions without scanning.

The multi-layered foils were fixed on top of an optical bench and the OCT probe head was moved across the foil at different speeds, ranging from 5 mm/s to 800 mm/s. The probing head was accelerated from its resting position (located on the left or right hand side) and the OCT measurements were performed in the center piece, where the velocity of the probe head was assumed to be constant. Subsequently the probing head was decelerated. The sample had an overall thickness of 290 μm and consisted of 10 different layers. Figure 2 shows a comparison of eight OCT images acquired at different speeds of the probing head, ranging from 5 mm/s to 800 mm/s. The images reveal that even at high speeds of the probing head the image quality allows for a distinction of the individual layers of the foil. The lateral size of the images has a speed dependency and can be calculated over $x = v/f$, where v is the probe head velocity in mm/s and f is the frame rate of the images (20 Hz). The image size in axial direction is 2.57 mm (measured in air).

Subsequently in-line measurements with the same OCT system were performed directly at a blown film extrusion line (Hosokawa Alpine), which is located at the Innovation Headquarter of Borealis Polyolefine in Linz, Austria. With this equipment it is possible to produce multi-layered multi-material foils consisting of up to seven individual layers. Throughout the experiments the overall foil thickness was varied between 30 μm and 200 μm, and the production speed was varied between 266 mm/s and 500 mm/s. The multi-layered foils consisted of layers of different materials (Borclear™ polypropylene, Borshape™ polyethylene, adhesion layer polymer, and EVOH - ethylene vinyl alcohol), where the EVOH layer was sandwiched between two layers of the other materials. Two exemplary OCT images acquired at a production speed of 500 mm/s are presented in Figure 3. Panel a) shows a foil with three layers and an overall thickness of 100 μm. Panel b) depicts two 100 μm thick foils with four layers each. Thickness measurements were performed on all images and showed a good accuracy with the values derived from the microscale measurements on the materials before entering the blown film extrusion line.

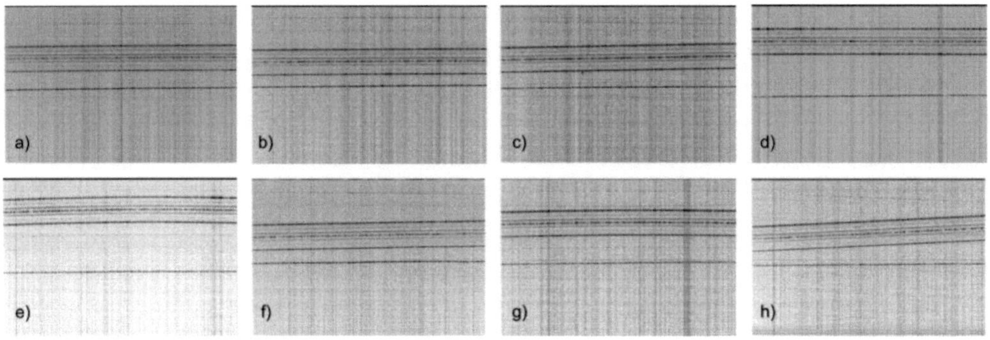

Figure 2. OCT images of multi-layered foils moving at different velocities of a) 5 mm/s; b) 10 mm/s; c) 20 mm/s; d) 50 mm/s; e) 100 mm/s; f) 200 mm/s; g) 300 mm/s; h) 800 mm/s. The image size in axial direction is 2.57 mm (measured in air). In lateral direction the image size has a speed dependency and is a) 0.25 mm; b) 0.5 mm; c) 1 mm; d) 2.5 mm; e) 5 mm; f) 10 mm; g) 15 mm; h) 40 mm [14].

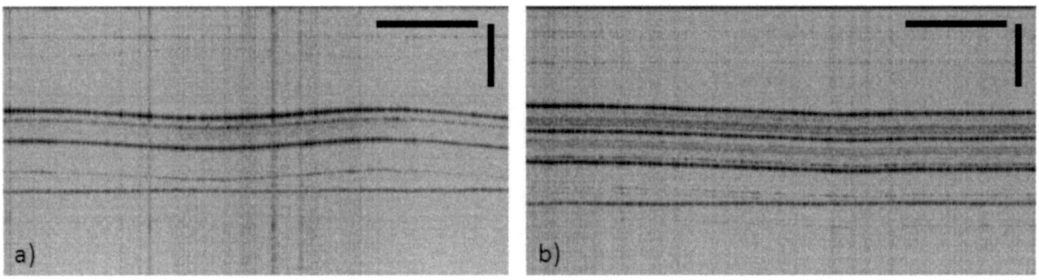

Figure 3. OCT cross-section images acquired in-line at the blow film extruder at a production speed of 500 mm/s; a) single foil with a thickness of 100 µm consisting of three different layers; b) double foil with 100 µm thickness each, consisting of four different layers. The black bars in the lateral and axial dimensions represent 5 mm and 0.3 mm, respectively.

These results showed the applicability of high speed and high resolution optical coherence tomography as a tool for the in-line quality control of multilayered foils. Future work could enhance the system performance towards a real in-line closed loop system. Real time imaging has already been shown with OCT [23], allowing therefore a real time observation of the sample directly during the production process. In this case a dedicated software analysis would provide the possibility to react on variations or inhomogeneities in the thickness of the individual foil layers. Therefore, with such a feed-back loop it should be possible to guarantee the highest quality of the product, to reduce waste, and hence to save resources.

3.2. OCT in plant photonics and for microstructure analysis in food

Until 2000 only a few reports on OCT applications in plant and food sciences were published. Most of them dealt with the layered structure of onions to highlight the applicability and capabilities of the respective OCT devices. The first ones publishing a dedicated report on this topic were Hettinger et al., who proposed optical coherence microscopy (OCM) as a technology for a rapid, in vivo, and non-destructive visualization of plants and plant cells [26]. Since then several general reports on the applicability of OCM/OCT on plant tissue have been published [27–31].

In 2004 Clements et al. reported a study on differences in the hull thickness in four different species of lupin seeds [32]. Lee et al. published work on disease detection in melon seeds [33] and apple leaves [34], proposing the technique as a suitable method for automated screening of viral infection in seeds and leaves, respectively. Detailed studies on the detection of defects, rots, and diseases in onions were published by Meglinski et al. [35] and Ford et al. [36].

An interesting kind of application is the use of OCT to analyze the microstructure of fresh pome fruit. Pome fruit like apples are often stored for several months, and the quality and thickness of the apple skin is one important parameter throughout the storing process [37], for it determines the protection of the apple against liquid and therefore weight loss. To show the ability of optical coherence tomography for the analysis and the control of wax layer thickness we performed OCT imaging sessions on Braeburn apples supplied by the Flanders Centre of Postharvest technology, Belgium. Figure 4 a) shows an OCT cross-section image acquired with an SD-OCT system similar to the one displayed in Figure 1. The image size is 4 x 1.25 mm^2 and several layers of the paring can clearly be distinguished. Other interesting features for the storage life of apples are the lenticels, which act as a bypass medium for the exchange of gases between the fruit flesh and the ambient. However, also bacteria and funguses can penetrate the fruit through the lenticels. Panels 4 b) and c) show OCT images of lenticels, as acquired with an ultra-high-resolution time-domain-OCT (UHR-TD-OCT) set-up. Panel 4 b) corresponds to a cross section with an image size of 3 x 0.3 mm^2. A lenticel is clearly visible in the lateral centre of the image, as indicated by the arrow. Panel 4 c) depicts an en-face image of an apple with an image size of 2 x 2 mm^2, as acquired with a UHR-TD-OCT system, showing the surface of the paring with a lenticel located in the centre. The fragmented appearance of this en-face image is due to the high axial resolution of the OCT set-up, which lies below two microns. Due to the curved shape of the apple, the flat OCT image plane does not fully coincide with the surface of the apple. As a result, in the image the upper left corner yields some bright surface reflections from the paring, whereas the lower part already shows some subsurface pores. Such pores are even better visible in panel 4 d), which has a size of 3 x 3 mm^2 and was acquired below the surface of another Braeburn apple. Once again, the fragmented appearance of the en-face OCT image is caused by the high axial resolution of the imaging system [38].

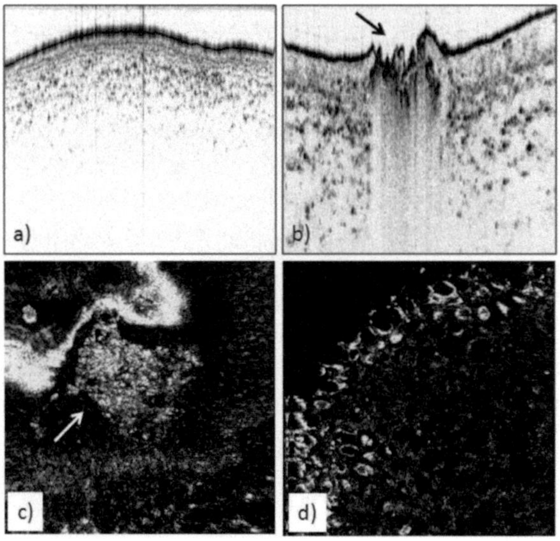

Figure 4. OCT images of Braeburn apples; a) Cross-section image acquired with an SD-OCT system. Image size: 4 x 1.25 mm^2; b) Cross-section image of a lenticel, acquired with a UHR-TD-OCT system. Image size: 3 x 0.3 mm^2; c) En-face OCT image of a lenticel (arrow), acquired with a UHR-TD-OCT set-up. Image size 2 x 2 mm^2; d) en-face OCT image of subsurface pores, acquired with the same system. Image size 3 x 3 mm^2 [38].

Another application of OCT in food science is the analysis of extruded breakfast cereals. In the case of extruded cereals the thickness and homogeneity of sugar coatings, as well as the pore size distribution of the uncoated cereals, are of special interest, since these parameters determine the rehydration properties and the crisp- and crunchiness, respectively. With the aid of OCT it is possible to analyze and monitor these quality indicators during the storage and production processes. Besides a simple analysis of the (sub)surface structures in extruded breakfast cereals it is also possible to study the dynamic rehydration process when immersing extruded breakfast cereals in a liquid like milk. As a specimen for this particular experiment we used coated extruded breakfast cereals provided by NESTEC. The cereals have a spherical shape with a mean diameter of 9 mm and a high surface roughness. They show a high porosity, and as a consequence in the OCT images only the topmost layer is visible. As a liquid we used semi-skimmed milk at room temperature (20°C). The experiments were performed with a Thorlabs TELESTO system. The extruded cereals were fixed on the bottom of a small cylindrical recipient, which was subsequently filled with milk up to approximately 80 % of the height of the cereal balls. 3D OCT images were recorded at a frame rate of 0.25 Hz while the cereal was soaked with milk. Figure 5 shows an OCT volume sequence for one such experiment. The volumes are ordered from a) – d) according to the progress in time during the experiment. Panel a) illustrates the surface of the cereals with no milk visible along the surface. In panel b) some first structural changes can be observed. In panels c) and d) more and more milk becomes apparent along the surface of the cereal ball, resulting in a reformation of the surface morphology. Also a shrinking of the height of the cereal becomes evident, as the structure of the extruded cereal ball is collapsing when being immersed in milk.

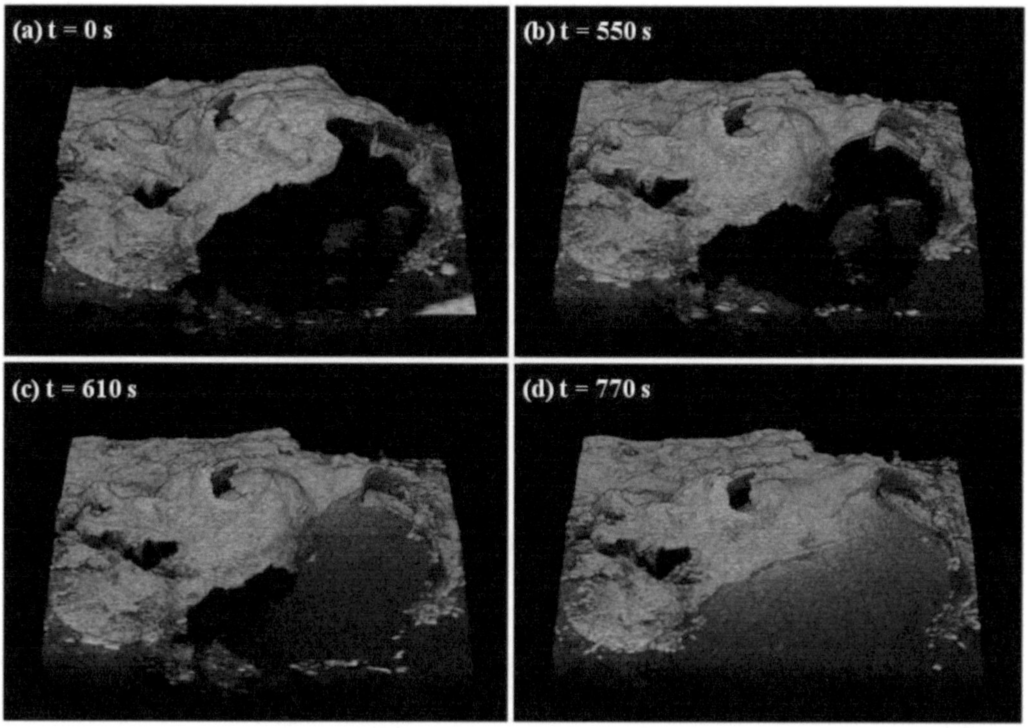

Figure 5. Temporal sequence of 3D OCT images showing the rehydration dynamics of extruded cereals in semi-skimmed milk. The images are ordered from (a) to (d) according to the progress in time. Image size: 4 × 4 × 2.5 mm^3.

The presented studies show the applicability of OCT as a tool in plant photonics and for the microstructure analysis in the food sciences.

3.3. Evaluation of laser induced (sub)surface structures

In many industrial processes there is a need for precise cutting or drilling in the micrometer range. Such cutting or drilling is often performed by ablating matter with the aid of picosecond or femtosecond laser light sources. In some recent publications OCT has been shown as a fast and non-destructive tool to assess the shape and depth of laser induced (sub)surface structures in a variety of different materials. The high sensitivity of OCT thereby allows the imaging of very steep edges, and OCT can also be used to give feedback on the optimum machining parameters. This can be done in a post-processing step, or in situ and in real-time during the machining process in order to give access to dynamic processes.

Webster et al. [39] reported in 2007 the use of light from the same high-power and broadband light source to perform both laser machining in stainless steel and direct observation of the written structures by means of OCT. The laser source was triggered in synchronism with the line scan device in the spectrometer and in this way it was possible to study the ablation dynamics via M-scans. In 2010 Wurm et al. [40] applied OCT to assess the depth and the width of laser drilled holes in a carbon fiber reinforced composite material by acquiring volume scans with subsequent application of a dedicated software algorithm. In the same year Webster et al. [16] used high speed M-mode OCT to detect relaxation effects between laser pulses in real-time. Furthermore they applied in situ M-mode OCT data to guide the cut into a lead zirconate titanate sample towards a certain target depth through a feedback loop controlling the number of laser pulses. A comparison of two OCT images acquired posterior and ex situ, one without (panel a) and one with (panel b) feedback, is depicted in Figure 6. Also Wiesner et al. [41] reported on in line process control in laser micromaching processes by means of OCT. Recently Goda et al. [42] showed the applicability of high throughput OCT with ~ 91 MHz axial scan rate for real-time monitoring of laser ablation dynamics caused by irradiation of a silicon sample with a mid-infrared laser pulse and a pulse width of 5 ns. With this ultra-high speed imaging system they even managed to acquire whole cross-sections within only 20 μs.

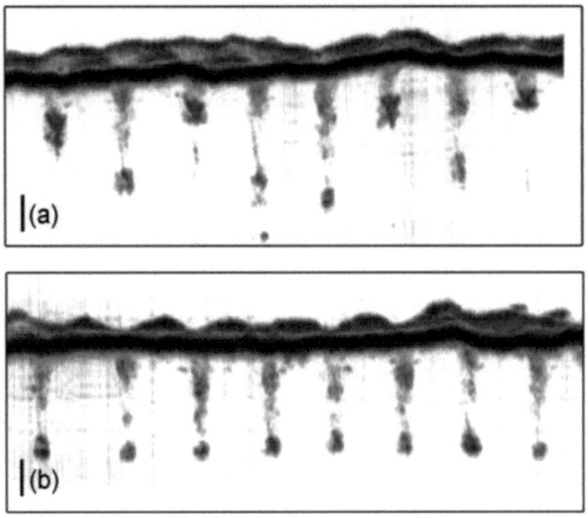

Figure 6. Side view of 3D surface topography of holes cut (a) without and (b) with feedback (B). Volumes above and below the surface correspond to air and steel, respectively. Scale bars are 100 μm (both axes). Reprinted from Paul J.L. Webster, Joe X.Z. Yu, Ben Y.C. Leung, Mitchell D. Anderson, Victor X.D. Yang, James M. Fraser, "*Coherent imaging of morphology change in laser percussion drilling*," Opt.Lett. 2010, *35*, 646-648, with permission from the Optical Society of America © 2010[16].

These recent studies highlight the high potential of OCT for the analysis of dynamic effects in laser micromachining and as a feedback tool to control the depth of the written structures.

3.4. Characterization of tablet coatings

A very recent application of OCT is the characterization of tablet coatings. Film coating is a widely used unit operation in the pharmaceutical industry for solid dosage form manufacturing, fulfilling different purposes ranging from aesthetic and trade marking issues to functionalized coatings, for taste masking, improved product stability, shelf life increase or

http://dx.doi.org/10.5772/53960

controlled release of the active pharmaceutical ingredient (API). In addition, functional coatings allow formulators to alter the initial drug release kinetics to be pH dependent by making it resistant to gastric juice through enteric coatings, i.e., controlled-release formulations. Alternatively, it is possible to retard the onset of the drug release by controlling the dissolution rate via semi-permeable membranes. Furthermore, active ingredients may be incorporated in the film layer [15].

Although coating processes have been used for many decades, there are still serious challenges, as there is a lack of understanding of how material and operating parameters impact product quality. Different problems can arise, such as picking (i.e., part of the film coating is pulled off one tablet and is deposited on another), twinning (i.e., two or more of the tablet cores are stuck together), orange peel (i.e., a roughened film due to spray drying), bridging (e.g., film coating lifts up out of the tablet logo), cracking (e.g., due to internal stresses in the film), coating inhomogeneity, and film thickness variations within a batch due to poor process and equipment design.

At the moment, there are many Process Analytical Technology (PAT) tools available, providing information about physicochemical product properties, ranging from the chemical composition or even the quantitative determination of the film coating thickness. Here, spectroscopic techniques like NIR and Raman were already demonstrated to be powerful tools for offline product characterization, as well as for in-line process monitoring. Combined with multivariate data analysis (MVDA), these methods enable for quantitative and non-invasive process monitoring and fulfill also most of the needs for robust and fast measurements.

However, these systems are often applied for characterizing the whole batch, where only averaged values for the film thickness are available from a moving tablet bed in a drum coater for instance. This value is a very good indicator for the overall process status, but provides little information about variations between single tablets, such as coating morphology and homogeneity. Even though well established quality control parameters, such as weight gain, indicate coating properties within specifications for the whole batch, no general conclusion can be drawn for the variation from tablet-to-tablet within a batch or the overall coating homogeneity of a single tablet. Hence, there is an increasing need for novel techniques, enabling accurate spatially (laterally and axially) resolved characterization of the coating. A comprehensive review on potential techniques fulfilling these requirements was given by Zeitler and Gladden [43], where X-ray computed microtomography (XμCT), magnetic resonance imaging (MRI), imaging at terahertz frequencies and OCT were evaluated and discussed for their informative value. These techniques can be considered as tomographic, i.e., allowing for a non-destructive three-dimensional investigation of dosage forms. In contrast to MRI and XμCT, OCT and terahertz pulsed imaging (TPI) are quite similar techniques and currently the only optical techniques used for non-destructive characterization of tablet coatings. Other studies on the application of OCT for the characterization of tablet coatings were published by Juuti et al. [44], Mauritz et al. [45], Zhong et al. [46] and Koller et al. [15].

In the work published by Koller et al. [15] OCT was utilized for a quantitative characterization of pharmaceutical tablet film coatings, sampled at different stages of an industrial drum spray coating process. OCT was selected from the above mentioned techniques due to its high axial and lateral resolution, which allows the investigation of very thin layers, due to its contact-free measurement properties, which is very important for curved surfaces and due to the high data acquisition rates for fast product characterization. The investigated tablets (round, biconvex Thrombo ASS 50 mg with an enteric coating of Eudragit® L30D-55) were sampled at 15 different stages (Lots) of the coating process, comprising tablets with a coating thickness ranging from uncoated to a target coating thickness of about 70 μm. The spray coating process was performed on a batch of approximately 1.2 million tablets using a BTC 400 perforated drum coater (L.B. Bohle Maschinen + Verfahren GmbH, Ennigerloh, Germany). From each sample set, five tablets were analyzed offline to get the statistical variation of the coating process. Besides the investigation with OCT in terms of layer thickness und homogeneity, tablet weight gain and tablet diameters were determined on a single-tablet level. Scanning electron microscopy (SEM) was applied on cracked tablets for referencing the coating thickness obtained with OCT.

Figure 7 shows a comparison between tablets of Lots 1, 7, 8, 9, 10, 11, 12, 14 and 15, as acquired with a spectral-domain OCT system similar to the one depicted in Figure 1. Details on the OCT system are available in Koller et al. [15]. The image size is 4.3 x 0.36 mm^2 with a resolution of 4.3 μm and < 4 μm in lateral and axial direction, respectively. The image acquisition rate was 1.5 images/s for the B-Scans (including display on screen). Due to the different resolutions, the images show different scales in lateral and axial direction. The illustrated coating thickness is represented by the optical path length, which is a function of the refractive index of the coating material ($n_{Eudragit} \approx 1.48$). Thus, an accurate determination of the coating thickness with the SD-OCT system is possible, as long as an appropriate contrast at the interfaces of the coating allows a clear discrimination between materials. The snapshots in Figure 7 are ordered from top to bottom according to the progress in the coating process, with Lot 1 representing a non-coated and Lot 15 a fully coated tablet. The increase in the coating thickness is clearly evident in the images. This highlights the potential of OCT, as even very thin layers at the beginning of the coating process can be analyzed. The arrows indicate defects in the coating or the underlying bulk material. These may result from inclusions of air during the coating process or density variations leading to increased light scattering. The features visible below the coating are caused by photons back-scattered from the substrate material. When using an OCT system working at longer wavelengths (e.g. 1300 nm) a deeper penetration into the substrate should be possible, however at the cost of a lower axial resolution.

With the results from the studies performed so far OCT turned out to be a very powerful tool for the characterization of tablet coatings.

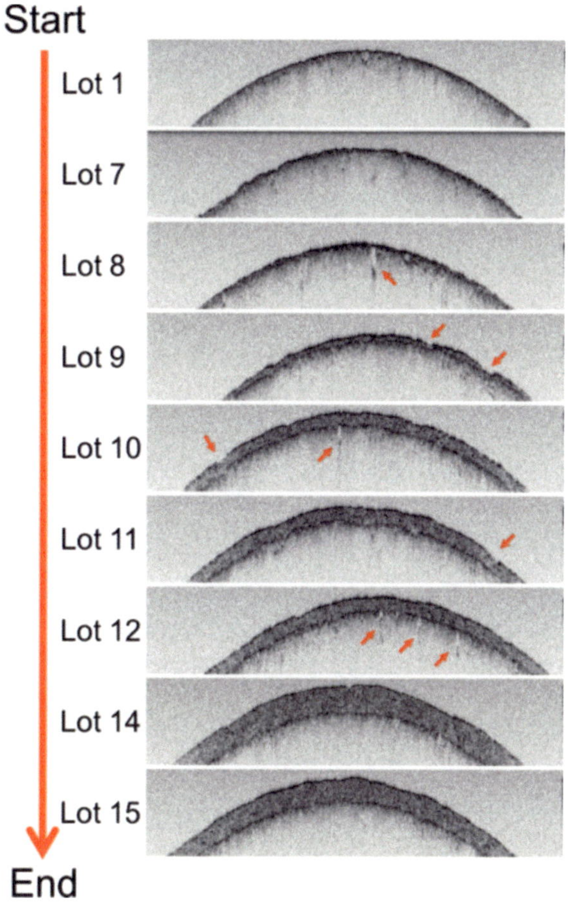

Figure 7. SD-OCT B-Scan images of tablets from different stages of the coating process. The image size is 4.3 x 0.36 mm^2 (measured in air) with a resolution of 4.3 μm and <4 μm in lateral and axial direction, respectively. Reprinted from Koller, D.M.; Hannesschläger, G.; Leitner, M.; Khinast, J.G. Non-destructive analysis of tablet coatings with optical coherence tomography. *European Journal of Pharmaceutical Sciences* 2011, *44*, 142–148, with permission from Elsevier © 2011 [15].

3.5. Evaluation of structural changes in materials

Many materials undergo structural changes during the production process or during their lifecycle. Examples include hardening, cooling or heating phases, or changes due to mechanical load or stress. OCT, and especially the functional extension of polarization sensitive OCT (PS-OCT), is a fast, fully contactless, and non-destructive approach to monitor and evaluate such processes. PS-OCT gives access to the birefringence of the sample and additional measurements of full Stokes vectors and Mueller matrices, as well as the simultaneous determination of intensity, retardation and orientation of the optical axes have been reported. A review on PS-OCT was published by de Boer et al. [47]. Reports on applications of PS-OCT in the field of NDT have been published, among others, in [12,13,21,48–55].

For a thorough review on applications of PS-OCT in the field of NDT the reader is referred to Chapter by Dr. Bettina Heise.

3.6. Other applications of OCT in NDTE

Besides the applications introduced so far, over the past few years OCT has also been applied to a vast variety of different samples and materials. For example several groups focused their efforts on the characterization of artwork, with a recent review on this topic having been published by Targowski et al. [22].

Especially the group around Myllylä in Oulu, Finland, is heavily engaged in the application of OCT for NDT. Over the last years they have applied OCT for the characterization of paper [56–59], printed electronics circuits [19,60] and also used OCT as a method for the characterization of wettability [61].

OCT can also be used to detect forgery in ancient jade [62] or banknotes [63], or the security thread in valuable documents [64]. A similar application is the one reported by Ju et al. for the evaluation and identification of pearls [65].

Furthermore, over the past few years OCT has been introduced as a tool to characterize and investigate samples, like e.g., organic solar cells [17], aerospace materials [66], light emitting diodes [67], periodically poled ferroelectrics [68], wet pad surfaces in chemical mechanical polishing processes [69], embedded micro channels in alumina ceramics [70], and even to study boiling phenomena [71].

4. Summary and outlook

In this chapter some applications of optical coherence tomography in non-destructive testing were presented and discussed. After an introduction to the technique of OCT and some considerations related to its use in non-destructive testing, a brief overview on the development of applications of OCT in the field of NDT was given. Special emphasis was paid to recent reports on topics like the characterization of multi-layered foils, studies on plant photonics and the microstructure in foods, the characterization of laser induced (sub)surface structures, and the determination of coating thickness in pharmaceutical tablets. In the end a brief overview on other NDT-related applications of OCT was provided.

With respect to the strong increase in the number of research groups working on OCT applications outside the field of biomedicine it is to be expected that the number of publications will rise drastically within the next few years. New applications for lab based and desktop OCT devices will be found, helping to better understand a wide variety of material systems and processes. On the other hand, so far the number of reports on the use of OCT in industrial environments and for the in situ and real-time monitoring of industrial processes is still scarce. However, some first and very promising reports pointing into this direction were reviewed in this chapter, triggering the demand for faster and more robust OCT devices in the future.

http://dx.doi.org/10.5772/53960

Acknowledgements

Financial support is gratefully acknowledged from the European Union (project FP7-226783 – InsideFood; The opinions expressed in this document do by no means reflect the official opinion of the European Union or its representatives), the „K-Project for Non-Destructive Testing and Tomography" supported by the COMET-program of the Austrian Research Promotion Agency (FFG), Grant No. 820492, the European Regional Development Fund (EFRE) in the framework of the EU-program REGIO 13, and the federal state of Upper Austria is gratefully acknowledged.

Author details

Alexandra Nemeth, Günther Hannesschläger, Elisabeth Leiss-Holzinger, Karin Wiesauer and Michael Leitner

*Address all correspondence to: michael.leitner@recendt.at

Research Center for Non-Destructive Testing GmbH, Linz, Austria

References

[1] Huang, D.; Swanson, E.A.; Lin, C.P.; Schuman, J.S.; Stinson, W.G.; Chang, W.; Hee; Flotte, T.; Gregory, K.; Puliafito, C.A.; et al. Optical coherence tomography. Science 1991, 254, 1178–1181.

[2] Drexler, W.; Morgner, U.; Kärtner, F.X.; Pitris, C.; Boppart, S.A.; Li, X.D.; Ippen, E.P.; Fujimoto, J.G. In vivo ultrahigh-resolution optical coherence tomography. Opt. Lett. 1999, 24, 1221–1223.

[3] Colston, B.; Sathyam, U.; DaSilva, L.; Everett, M.; Stroeve, P.; Otis, L. Dental OCT. Opt. Express 1998, 3, 230–238.

[4] Podoleanu, A.; Rogers, J.; Jackson, D.; Dunne, S. Three dimensional OCT images from retina and skin. Opt. Express 2000, 7, 292–298.

[5] Jang, I.-K.; Bouma, B.E.; Kang, D.-H.; Park, S.-J.; Park, S.-W.; Seung, K.-B.; Choi, K.-B.; Shishkov, M.; Schlendorf, K.; Pomerantsev, E.; et al. Visualization of coronary atherosclerotic plaques in patients using optical coherence tomography: comparison with intravascular ultrasound. Journal of the American College of Cardiology 2002, 39, 604–609.

[6] Jenkins, M.W.; Duke, A.R.; Gu, S.; Doughman, Y.; Chiel, H.J.; Fujioka, H.; Watanabe, M.; Jansen, E.D.; Rollins, A.M. Optical pacing of the embryonic heart. Nat Photon 2010, 4, 623–626.

[7] Swanson, E.A.; Hee, M.R.; Tearney, G.J.; Fujimoto, J.G. Application of optical coherence tomography in nondestructive evaluation of material microstructure. In Lasers and Electro-Optics, 1996. CLEO '96., 1996, pp. 326–327.

[8] Bashkansky, M.; Battle, P.R.; Duncan, M.D.; Kahn, M.; Reintjes, J. Subsurface Defect Detection in Ceramics Using an Optical Gated Scatter Reflectometer. Journal of the American Ceramic Society 1996, 79, 1397–1400.

[9] Bashkansky, M.; Duncan, M.D.; Kahn, M.; Lewis III, D.; Reintjes, J. Subsurface defect detection in ceramics by high-speed high-resolution optical coherent tomography. Opt. Lett. 1997, 22, 61–63.

[10] Duncan, M.; Bashkansky, M.; Reintjes, J. Subsurface defect detection in materialsusing optical coherence tomography. Opt. Express 1998, 2, 540–545.

[11] Wiesauer, K.; Pircher, M.; Götzinger, E.; Bauer, S.; Engelke, R.; Ahrens, G.; Grützner, G.; Hitzenberger, C.; Stifter, D. En-face scanning optical coherence tomography with ultra-high resolution for material investigation. Opt. Express 2005, 13, 1015–1024.

[12] Wiesauer, K.; Pircher, M.; Goetzinger, E.; Hitzenberger, C.K.; Engelke, R.; Ahrens, G.; Gruetzner, G.; Stifter, D. Transversal ultrahigh-resolution polarization-sensitive optical coherence tomography for strain mapping in materials. Opt. Express 2006, 14, 5945–5953.

[13] Stifter, D. Beyond Biomedicine: A Review of Alternative Applications And Developments For Optical Coherence Tomography. Applied Physics B 2007, 88, 337–357.

[14] Hannesschläger, G.; Nemeth, A.; Hofer, C.; Goetzloff, C.; Reussner, J.; Wiesauer, K.; Leitner, M. Optical coherence tomography as a tool for non destructive quality control of multi-layered foils. In Proceedings of the 6th NDT in Progress 2011, International Workshop of NDT Experts, Prag, 10.09-12.09.2011, 2011, pp. Paper 7.

[15] Koller, D.M.; Hannesschläger, G.; Leitner, M.; Khinast, J.G. Non-destructive analysis of tablet coatings with optical coherence tomography. European Journal of Pharmaceutical Sciences 2011, 44, 142–148.

[16] Webster, P.J.L.; Yu, J.X.Z.; Leung, B.Y.C.; Anderson, M.D.; Yang, V.X.D.; Fraser, J.M. In situ 24 kHz coherent imaging of morphology change in laser percussion drilling. Opt. Lett 2010, 35, 646-648.

[17] Thrane, L.; Jørgensen, T.M.; Jørgensen, M.; Krebs, F.C. Application of optical coherence tomography (OCT) as a 3-dimensional imaging technique for roll-to-roll coated polymer solar cells. Solar Energy Materials and Solar Cells 2012, 97, 181–185.

[18] Alarousu, E.; Krehut, L.; Prykäri, T.; Myllylä, R. Study on the use of optical coherence tomography in measurements of paper properties. Measurement Science and Technology 2005, 16, 1131.

[19] Czajkowski, J.; Prykäri, T.; Alarousu, E.; Palosaari, J.; Myllylä, R. Optical coherence tomography as a method of quality inspection for printed electronics products. Optical Review 2010, 17, 257–262.

[20] Stifter, D.; Leiss-Holzinger, E.; Major, Z.; Baumann, B.; Pircher, M.; Götzinger, E.; Hitzenberger, C.K.; Heise, B. Dynamic optical studies in materials testing with spectral-domain polarization-sensitive optical coherence tomography. Optics Express 2010, 18, 25712–25725.

[21] Targowski, P.; Iwanicka, M. Optical Coherence Tomography: its role in the non-invasive structural examination and conservation of cultural heritage objects - a review. Applied Physics A: Materials Science & Processing 2012, 106, 265–277.

[22] van der Jeught, S.; Bradu, A.; Podoleanu, A.G. Real-time resampling in Fourier domain optical coherence tomography using a graphics processing unit. J. Biomed. Opt. 2010, 15, 30511–3.

[23] Chen, Z.; Milner, T.E.; Dave, D.; Nelson, J.S. Optical Doppler tomographic imaging of fluid flow velocity in highly scattering media. Opt. Lett. 1997, 22, 64–66.

[24] Pircher, M.; Götzinger, E.; Leitgeb, R.; Fercher, A.; Hitzenberger, C. Measurement and imaging of water concentration in human cornea with differential absorption optical coherence tomography. Opt. Express 2003, 11, 2190–2197.

[25] Hettinger, J.W.; La Mattozzi, M.P. de; Myers, W.R.; Williams, M.E.; Reeves, A.; Parsons, R.L.; Haskell, R.C.; Petersen, D.C.; Wang, R.; Medford, J.I. Optical Coherence Microscopy. A Technology for Rapid, in Vivo, Non-Destructive Visualization of Plants and Plant Cells. Plant Physiology 2000, 123, 3–16.

[26] Reeves, A.; Parsons, R.L.; Hettinger, J.W.; Medford, J.I. In vivo three-dimensional imaging of plants with optical coherence microscopy. Journal of Microscopy 2002, 208, 177-189.

[27] Sapozhnikova, V.V.; Kamenskii, V.A.; Kuranov, R.V. Visualization of Plant Tissues by Optical Coherence Tomography. Russian Journal of Plant Physiology 2003, 50, 282–286.

[28] Kutis, I.S.; Sapozhnikova, V.V.; Kuranov, R.V.; Kamenskii, V.A. Study of the Morphological and Functional State of Higher Plant Tissues by Optical Coherence Microscopy and Optical Coherence Tomography. Russian Journal of Plant Physiology 2005, 52, 559–564.

[29] Boccara, M.; Schwartz, W.; Guiot, E.; Vidal, G.; Paepe, R. de; Dubois, A.; Boccara, A.-C. Early chloroplastic alterations analysed by optical coherence tomography during a harpin-induced hypersensitive response. The Plant Journal 2007, 50, 338–346.

[30] Loeb, G.; Barton, J.K. Imaging botanical subjects with optical coherence tomography: a feasibility study, 2008.

[31] Clements, J.C.; Zvyagin, A.V.; Silva, K.K.M.B.D.; Wanner, T.; Sampson, D.D.; Cowling, W.A. Optical coherence tomography as a novel tool for non-destructive measurement of the hull thickness of lupin seeds. Plant Breeding 2004, 123, 266-270.

[32] Lee, C.; Lee, S.-Y.; Kim, J.-Y.; Jung, H.-Y.; Kim, J. Optical Sensing Method for Screening Disease in Melon Seeds by Using Optical Coherence Tomography. Sensors 2011, 11, 9467-9477.

[33] Lee, C.-H.; Lee, S.-Y.; Jung, H.-Y.; Kim, J.-H. The Application of Optical Coherence Tomography in the Diagnosis of Marssonina Blotch in Apple Leaves. J. Opt. Soc. Korea 2012, 16, 133-140.

[34] Meglinski, I.; Buranachai, C.; Terry, L. Plant photonics: application of optical coherence tomography to monitor defects and rots in onion. Laser Physics Letters 2010, 7, 307-310.

[35] Ford, H.D.; Tatam, R.P.; Landahl, S.; Terry, L.A. Investigation of disease in stored onions using optical coherence tomography. In IV International Conference Postharvest Unlimited 2011, pp. 247–254.

[36] Veraverbeke, E.A.; van Bruaene, N.; van Oostveldt, P.; Nicolaï, B.M. Non destructive analysis of the wax layer of apple Malus domestica by means of confocal laser scanning microscopy. Planta 2001, 213, 525–533.

[37] Leitner, M.; Hannesschläger, G.; Saghy, A.; Nemeth, A.; Chassagne-Berces, S.; Chanvrier, H.; Herremans, E.; Verlinden, B. Optical coherence tomography for quality control and microstructure analysis in food. In ICEF Athens, 22.-26.05.2011, 2011.

[38] Webster, P.J.L.; Muller, M.S.; Fraser, J.M. High speed in situ depth profiling of ultrafast micromachining. Opt. Express 2007, 15, 14967-14972.

[39] Wurm, M.; Hofer, C.; Traxler, H.; Zabernig, A.; Harrer, B. Vermessung der Laserbohrungen in faserverstärktem Graphit mittels Optischer Kohärenztomographie. In Industrielle Computertomographie, Wels, 27.-29.09.2010, 2010, pp. 133–140.

[40] Wiesner, M.; Ihlemann, J.; Muller, H.H.; Lankenau, E.; Huttmann, G. Optical coherence tomography for process control of laser micromachining. Rev. Sci. Instrum. 2010, 81, 33705–7.

[41] Goda, K.; Fard, A.; Malik, O.; Fu, G.; Quach, A.; Jalali, B. High-throughput optical coherence tomography at 800 nm. Opt. Express 2012, 20, 19612–19617.

[42] Zeitler, J.A.; Gladden, L.F. In-vitro tomography and non-destructive imaging at depth of pharmaceutical solid dosage forms: Special Issue: Solid State and Solid Dosage Forms. European Journal of Pharmaceutics and Biopharmaceutics 2009, 71, 2–22.

[43] Juuti, M.; Tuononen, H.; Prykäri, T.; Kontturi, V.; Kuosmanen, M.; Alarousu, E.; Ketolainen, J.; Myllylä, R.; Peiponen, K. Optical and terahertz measurement techniques for flat-faced pharmaceutical tablets: a case study of gloss, surface roughness and

bulk properties of starch acetate tablets. Measurement Science and Technology 2009, 20, 15301.

[44] Mauritz, J.M.A.; Morrisby, R.S.; Hutton, R.S.; Legge, C.H.; Kaminski, C.F. Imaging pharmaceutical tablets with optical coherence tomography. J. Pharm. Sci. 2010, 99, 385–391.

[45] Zhong, S.; Shen, Y.-C.; Ho, L.; May, R.K.; Zeitler, J.A.; Evans, M.; Taday, P.F.; Pepper, M.; Rades, T.; Gordon, K.C.; et al. Non-destructive quantification of pharmaceutical tablet coatings using terahertz pulsed imaging and optical coherence tomography. Optics and Lasers in Engineering 2011, 49, 361–365.

[46] Boer, J.F. de; Milner, T.E. Review of polarization sensitive optical coherence tomography and Stokes vector determination. J. Biomed. Opt. 2002, 7, 359–371.

[47] Oh, J.-T.; Kim, S.-W. Polarization-sensitive optical coherence tomography for photoelasticity testing of glass/epoxy composites. Opt. Express 2003, 11, 1669–1676.

[48] Stifter, D.; Burgholzer, P.; Höglinger, O.; Götzinger, E.; Hitzenberger, C.K. Polarisation-sensitive optical coherence tomography for material characterisation and strain-field mapping. Applied Physics A: Materials Science & Processing 2003, 76, 947–951.

[49] Wiesauer, K.; Dufau, A.D.S.; Götzinger, E.; Pircher, M.; Hitzenberger, C.K.; Stifter, D. Non-destructive quantification of internal stress in polymer materials by polarisation sensitive optical coherence tomography. Acta Materialia 2005, 53, 2785–2791.

[50] Wiesauer, K.; Pircher, M.; Götzinger, E.; Hitzenberger, C.K.; Oster, R.; Stifter, D. Investigation of glass–fibre reinforced polymers by polarisation-sensitive, ultra-high resolution optical coherence tomography: Internal structures, defects and stress. Composites Science and Technology 2007, 67, 3051–3058.

[51] Engelke, R.; Ahrens, G.; Arndt-Staufenbiehl, N.; Kopetz, S.; Wiesauer, K.; Löchel, B.; Schröder, H.; Kastner, J.; Neyer, A.; Stifter, D.; et al. Investigations on possibilities of inline inspection of high aspect ratio microstructures. Microsystem Technologies 2007, 13, 319–325.

[52] Wiesauer, K.; Pircher, M.; Gtzinger, E.; Hitzenberger, C.K.; Engelke, R.; Grtzner, G.; Ahrens, G.; Oster, R.; Stifter, D. Measurement of structure and strain by transversal ultra-high resolution polarisation-sensitive optical coherence tomography. Insight - Non-Destructive Testing and Condition Monitoring 2007, 49, 275–278.

[53] Heise, B.; Wiesauer, K.; Götzinger, E.; Pircher, M.; Hitzenberger, C.K.; Engelke, R.; Ahrens, G.; Grützner, G.; Stifter, D. Spatially Resolved Stress Measurements in Materials With Polarisation-Sensitive Optical Coherence Tomography: Image Acquisition and Processing Aspects. Strain 2010, 46, 61–68.

[54] Leiss-Holzinger, E.; Cakmak, U.D.; Heise, B.; Bouchot, J.L.; Klement, E.P.; Leitner, M.; Stifter, D.; Major, Z. Evaluation of structural change and local strain distribution in polymers comparatively imaged by FFSA and OCT techniques. eXPRESS Polymer Letters 2012, 6, 249–256.

[55] Alarousu, E.; Krehut, L.; Prykäri, T.; Myllylä, R. Study on the use of optical coherence tomography in measurements of paper properties. Measurement Science and Technology 2005, 16, 1131.

[56] Fabritius, T.; Myllylä, R. Liquid sorption investigation of porous media by optical coherence tomography. Journal of Physics D: Applied Physics 2006, 39, 4668.

[57] Fabritius, T.; Myllylä, R. Investigation of swelling behaviour in strongly scattering porous media using optical coherence tomography. Journal of Physics D: Applied Physics 2006, 39, 2609.

[58] Prykäri, T.; Czajkowski, J.; Alarousu, E.; Myllylä, R. Optical coherence tomography as an accurate inspection and quality evaluation technique in paper industry. Optical Review 2010, 17, 218–222.

[59] Czajkowski, J.; Fabritius, T.; Ulański, J.; Marszałek, T.; Gazicki-Lipman, M.; Nosal, A.; Śliż, R.; Alarousu, E.; Prykäri, T.; Myllylä, R.; et al. Ultra-high resolution optical coherence tomography for encapsulation quality inspection. Applied Physics B: Lasers and Optics 2011, 105, 649–657.

[60] Fabritius, T.; Myllylä, R.; Makita, S.; Yasuno, Y. Wettability characterization method based on optical coherence tomography imaging. Opt. Express 2010, 18, 22859–22866.

[61] Chang, S.; Mao, Y.; Chang, G.; Flueraru, C. Jade detection and analysis based on optical coherence tomography images. Optical Engineering 2010, 49, 63602.

[62] Choi, W.-J.; Min, G.-H.; Lee, B.-H.; Eom, J.-H.; Kim, J.-W. Counterfeit Detection Using Characterization of Safety Feature on Banknote with Full-field Optical Coherence Tomography. J. Opt. Soc. Korea 2010, 14, 316–320.

[63] Fujiwara, K.; Matoba, O. High-speed cross-sectional imaging of valuable documents using common-path swept-source optical coherence tomography. Appl. Opt. 2011, 50, H165.

[64] Ju, M.J.; Lee, S.J.; Min, E.J.; Kim, Y.; Kim, H.Y.; Lee, B.H. Evaluating and identifying pearls and their nuclei by using optical coherence tomography. Opt. Express 2010, 18, 13468–13477.

[65] Liu, P.; Groves, R.M.; Benedictus, R. Quality assessment of aerospace materials with optical coherence tomography 2012, 84300I.

[66] Cho, N.H.; Jung, U.; Kim, S.; Kim, J. Non-Destructive Inspection Methods for LEDs Using Real-Time Displaying Optical Coherence Tomography. Sensors 2012, 12, 10395-10406.

[67] Pei, S.-C.; Ho, T.-S.; Tsai, C.-C.; Chen, T.-H.; Ho, Y.; Huang, P.-L.; Kung, A.H.; Huang, S.-L. Non-invasive characterization of the domain boundary and structure properties of periodically poled ferroelectrics. Opt. Express 2011, 19, 7153–7160.

[68] Choi, W.J.; Jung, S.P.; Shin, J.G.; Yang, D.; Lee, B.H. Characterization of wet pad surface in chemical mechanical polishing (CMP) process with full-field optical coherence tomography (FF-OCT). Opt. Express 2011, 19, 13343–13350.

[69] Su, R.; Kirillin, M.; Ekberg, P.; Roos, A.; Sergeeva, E.; Mattsson, L. Optical coherence tomography for quality assessment of embedded microchannels in alumina ceramic. Opt. Express 2012, 20, 4603–4618.

[70] Meissner, S.; Herold, J.; Kirsten, L.; Schneider, C.; Koch, E. 3D optical coherence tomography as new tool for microscopic investigations of nucleate boiling on heated surfaces. International Journal of Heat and Mass Transfer 2012, 55, 5565–5569.